# Hello Gorgeous!

# Hello Gorgeous!
## A Journey of
## Faith, Love and Hope

By Kim and Mike Becker

HELLO GORGEOUS!
A Journey of Love, Faith and Hope

10 9 8 7 6 5 4 3 2 1

ISBN 978-0-9833586-4-0

Library of Congress Control Number 2011939707

Published by
**Corby Books**
A Division of Corby Publishing LP
P.O. Box 93
Notre Dame, Indiana 46556
(574) 784-3482
www.corbypublishing.com

Manufactured in the United States of America

*To Bring the Promise of Beauty and Vitality Back into*
*The Hearts of All Those Touched by Cancer*

*This book is dedicated to God, for giving us this amazing project that we, alone, could never have thought up nor moved forward. And to our 9-year-old son, Seth Michael, for his patience, enthusiasm and for giving us our first dollar for this project from his own money when he was 4. Thank you both.*

*And to all the Gorgeous Women that it has been our great pleasure to surprise, hug, make over, hug, cry with and hug again. May all of you win your battle, find your path and live happy and healthy to 90 years old.*

*And may the last words you hear be "Hello Gorgeous!"*

# Introduction

HELLO GORGEOUS! OF HOPE, INC. is a non-profit organization that provides complimentary, professional makeovers and cosmetic education to all women battling all cancers. These services are provided in either a 34' RV redesigned as a mobile DaySpa or in one of the partnering Affiliate Salons in Indiana and other surrounding states.

These are surprise makeovers. All women served by our program are nominated by family or friends and their nominations are looked over by a selection committee, which chooses the women to be helped based on merit, need and availability.

Once chosen, arrangements are made with the individual nominating the woman with cancer to have her at a prearranged location or salon for the event. We show up unannounced and:

- surprise them with candy, flowers and a big "Hello Gorgeous!"
- treat them to spa services including manicure, pedicure and facial;
- give a hair consultation and makeup application;
- many times, gift them with a new clothing outfit;
- and many times, publicly reveal the woman with her "new look" to a prearranged, gathered

group of her family and friends.

We have found that the services and education we provide can allow these women a positive anchor during their battle with cancer and a *mending event*; physical services that have been proven, many times, to be restorative to a woman's mind and spirit, and also cosmetic techniques that are education-specific to the effects of their cancer treatments and the side-effects of those treatments. We pamper them for a day and instruct them how to help conceal the physical damages to their looks with specialized products and techniques that we can provide.

Simply stated, our mission is to provide cosmetic aid and education to those battling cancer. We strive to strengthen the knowledge of cancer patients and survivors concerning their hair styling, hair substitution, skin care and cosmetic techniques that will allow them to return to their jobs, their families, their friends and to the general public with confidence and courage. We want to help them step back into the world with some of that confidence and poise taken from them by the disease that they struggle to conquer.

This is the mission and passion of Hello Gorgeous! of HOPE, Inc.

# FAITH

# faith (fay-TH)

*n.*

1. Confident belief in the truth, value and trustworthiness of a person, idea or thing.
2. Belief that does not rest on logical proof or material evidence.
3. Loyalty to a person or thing.
4. A set of principles or beliefs.

# One Definition of FAITH

FOLLOWING A CALLING IS A DIFFICULT THING. Those who rise to that challenge can be looked upon as eccentric and (let's face it) a little deranged. It takes faith to follow a calling, but even more faith to help those who do. Our family and friends are our most loyal volunteers and we can never thank them enough for all the help and support they show us every day. We would like to thank our parents, Janice and Guy Chapman and John Becker, for the endless love and support they give to us every day. To our siblings and their families: Amy and Pat Hechlinski, Tina and Sean Fredericks, Trisha and Dan Greenlee, and Maria and Jeremy Becker-Yates for their endless support and confidence. To our Aunt Sue Maggio, whom we had the honor of serving as a Gorgeous Woman during her own battle with cancer, for her help with the Affiliate Salon program and her prayers. To our cousin Mary Woolling for her knowledge of the book publishing world and her constant praise and encouragement for this book project and for Hello Gorgeous! itself. To Mark and Jen Durocher for being the voice of Hello Gorgeous! at our premiere events and for their endless talents. To Mary Jo

3

Smith for her invaluable help transcribing all of these wonderful stories. To Bob and Valerie Simmons of A Thousand Words Photography, Classic Image Photography and the other talented photographers who have donated their time and talents to our cause to document and depict the images of these beautiful and precious Gorgeous Women.

And to those of our family who have gone before us: Jeanine Becker (Mike's mother), Larry Scanlan (Kim's father) and Jean Bowersox—for the love you always gave and for all you taught us.

I need to thank my sister, my assistant, my Affiliate Salon Training instructor and one of our Creative Directors of Hello Gorgeous, Trisha Greenlee, who has been with Mike and I

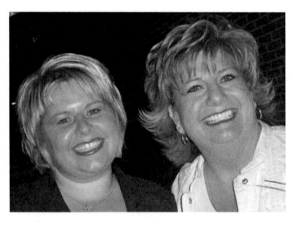

on this adventure since Hello Gorgeous! began. I don't think Hello Gorgeous! would exist without her. Thanks, Trisha.

We need to thank the members of our talented **Executive Team:** Dan and Trisha Greenlee and Thad and Elissa Schmidt. Their diverse and passionate talents, their gifts of ideas and counsel, and their sacrifice of time with their families to participate in this project will always be one of our greatest resources. We love you all.

Thank you also to our army of **Gorgeous Volunteers**. There are literally too many amazing people to mention, but especially people like Kelly Taddeo, Julie Chrobot and

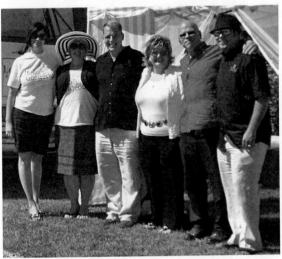

The Team: Elissa, Trisha, Thad, Kim, Mike and Dan

Chris Sacha, who help to further this cause in so many ways; whether they spend a single Saturday sweating with us as we work a Notre Dame Stadium concession stand or spend many months with the details of a large fundraiser. These selfless individuals see the value of Hello Gorgeous! and always step out in faith to help.

To all our generous Corporate Sponsors who understand the need for our services and who donate their support for the sake and care of our Gorgeous Women. May your kindness and sacrifices return to you tenfold, blessing you in the years to come.

To Jim Langford of Corby Books, Lakeville, Indiana, for his love of our book, his infectious laugh, his passion for his industry and for his 40 years experience in the publishing industry that made this book possible. Tim Carroll of

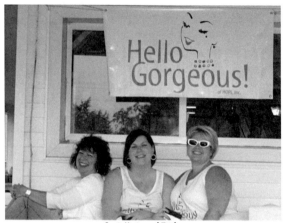
Suzi, Katie and Trisha

Corby Books lent us his design and printing expertise with enthusiasm and good spirit.

And, finally, to all of you. May your time spent within these pages allow your hearts and minds to be opened to the plight of these amazing women diagnosed with cancer. Thank you for helping us to help all of them. God Bless.

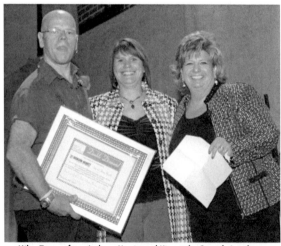
Mike, Tammy from Jackson Hewitt and Kim at the Comedy Luncheon

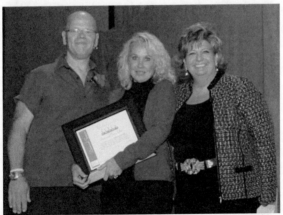

Hello Gorgeous!

# Special Thank You

THIS IS A SPECIAL THANK YOU to some remarkable individuals and their companies that have stepped forward in faith to supply Hello Gorgeous! with the products and equipment to fulfill our mission for our women battling cancer. Their vision allows us to have purpose and impact and we are deeply indebted to them.

Mike, Terry from Sella Skincare and Kim at the 2010 Comedy Luncheon

To Dennis, Terri and Anthony of Sella All-Natural Skincare of Chicago for their amazing promise in donating their world-class nanotechnology skin care to each Gorgeous Woman helped through our program.

To Dan of Graham Beauty Supply for approaching his company to donate all the key sanitary spa components used during the gorgeous visits to protect our women battling cancer from infection during their services.

To the Paula Young Wig Company for donating all the wigs and hats for every visit and the promise through their foundation to continue doing so.

To Jason, Melissa and the entire crew from Minerva Beauty Equipment of Duluth, Georgia, for donating brand new spa equipment for a DaySpa-on-wheels, 800 miles away from their location, sight unseen, as a result of a single phone call from Hello Gorgeous!

There are so many other generous people who have stepped forward to help us through their products and services. People complain that there is less charity and caring in this world, but the best of humanity can be found by showing the best of humanity in yourself. And it has always surrounded Hello Gorgeous! Words cannot express our gratitude.

**"Faith is reason grown courageous."**

*– Sherwood Eddy*

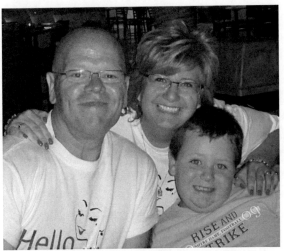

Hello Gorgeous!

# Our Story

Kim and Mike Becker (and son, Seth), Founders of Hello Gorgeous!

KIM AND MIKE BECKER began Hello Gorgeous! in September 2005 as a calling. Kim has been a hairdresser for 25 years and a salon owner for ten years. She has trained with Pivot Point International in Chicago, Haircolor USA in Miami, the Repechage Academy, Vidal Sassoon in London and has also been an educator for Jessica Cosmetics in Beverly Hills and the Italian-based color line Framesi, where she trained other hair colorists on new color techniques and color formulations. Kim has been married to her BFF Mike for 18 years and has a 9-year-old son, Seth Michael, who is her pride and joy.

9

In 1997 Kim and Mike opened their own salon, which they grew into one of the largest full-service salons in South Bend, Indiana, at 3000 square feet, with ten stylists, five colorists, three nail technicians, an esthetician and two massage therapists. Mike earned his BA from Purdue University and spent 20 years as a corporate manager of hundreds of employees in all aspects of sales and service—the last eight years managing the salon as well.

After helping many of her clients, relatives and friends through their cosmetic challenges over the years during their cancer treatments, Kim began working with cancer patients in group settings to help them cope with drastic changes in their appearance, through the use of cosmetics and hair substitution. But in talking with these women, Kim realized that these women needed more and she needed to take it a step further.

Kim and Mike had owned their salon for ten years. They sold it and applied for their 501(c)(3) non-profit status in August 2005, still not knowing why they wanted to give up a successful salon for something untried. They attended the Chicago Midwest Beauty Show in March 2006 with nothing but their business cards and the knowledge of how many hundreds of women would benefit from this personalized service at the most challenging time in their lives. They have never looked back.

**"One with passion is better than
40 with just an interest."**

– *Tom Connellan*

Hello
Gorgeous!

# The Hello Gorgeous! Experience
## Or
## "You could answer the phone "Hello Gorgeous!" and it would make them smile."

WHEN WE FIRST STARTED HELLO GORGEOUS! we began serving these women from our salon in South Bend, Indiana; spa services, makeup, maybe a wig and lots of love. That worked for a few years—the visits were once a month, we had very few nominations at that time because we were relatively unknown in the community and our vision was still small and local. But our goal had always been to create a mobile salon, a rolling palace that could go to those women who were too ill to leave the area of their home or just unwilling because of their struggles with their appearance. We wanted a mobile day spa with every convenience you would find in a top salon, so that we could offer any service they might need, all in the comfort and anonymity of a private environment.

Through the grace of God and our diligent, creative and *endless* fundraising over the next three years, we were blessed to find and purchase our DaySpa: a 1995 Holiday Rambler RV that a handful of donated salon equipment, some very talented renovators and an interior decorator with a vision turned into the *Gorgeous Endeavor*, our rolling palace for our women battling cancer. The journey had truly begun.

11

This book is written about some of the women battling cancer that we have helped with our services. We call them

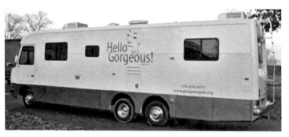

our "Gorgeous Women." And I thought I would start with the story of how we actually came to be called Hello Gorgeous!

My name is Kim Becker and my husband Michael and I started this organization in 2005 as a calling. We owned a full-service hair salon in South Bend, Indiana, for ten years. When we first thought to open the salon, my husband said to me, "I know what we should call the salon. We should call it 'Hello Gorgeous.'"

I promptly told him that was the stupidest thing I had ever heard in my entire life and that we were not calling it "Hello" anything! I had been an educator for a West Coast nail company many years before and had been very impressed by a salon there where I had given several classes. It was a beautiful and elegant A-frame building, all of glass, and they had served champagne and cheesecake to all their clients. It was called Cheveux, which meant "hair" in French, and I had always known that when I opened a salon I would call it that.

"No, no, it will be really cool," Mike said, "because every time you pick up the phone, if you greet the person on the other end with 'Hello Gorgeous!' it would make them smile." I told him that was dumb and we weren't doing it. The name was picked out!

We opened Cheveux and owned it for ten years. We grew the business quite a bit by the time we sold it. As in every business we had our ups and downs between employees, taxes, wages, utilities and repairs. But I found that I just could not find in the salon the complete fulfillment that I very much needed.

There was just something missing. There was an emptiness that I could not explain.

I thought that maybe there was something missing in me. So, I went to classes to further my education. I trained in Chicago and Miami and New York and I even went to Vidal Sassoon in London to train, which was one of my dreams. Still I never seemed to find the fulfillment I was looking for. I became an educator for the color line that we used in our salon at the time and I did a lot of traveling for them, teaching classes. Many of the salons where I demonstrated this particular color line were in downtown Chicago; top salons in the industry were asking for me as their instructor. Still I was not finding that fulfillment I was looking for.

I thought maybe a change would help. So we moved our salon across town, from one location to another, and tripled our size. We expanded our services and, over a few years, grew to 14 hair stations with stylists and colorists from beginner to master, massage rooms, tanning beds, nail and pedicure rooms, esthetics room and multiple office staff. We did constant promotions, like referral programs, product sales for holidays, back-to-school specials for product and services and "The Boss Is on Vacation" sales. We had *thousands* of clients and did a great business. Yes, it was coffee and mints, rather than champagne and cheesecake, but a wonderful salon nevertheless.

And still the emptiness was there. That is the only way I can describe it, just "an emptiness."

In 2005, on a trip back from Indianapolis, Indiana, Mike and I were talking as our son Seth slept in the back seat of the car. I talked with Mike about that same thing that I had felt for a year or more, that I just felt like there was something else that we should be doing, that I thought there was a higher purpose for us. Suddenly I looked at him and I said, "I know what we're supposed to do!" Mike's eyes got big and he listened intently as he drove because he too was kind of down on our salon. It had been so much work all the time, for so many years, and it seemed like we just couldn't get it to where we thought it should be. He was looking for a higher purpose as well.

"We're supposed to have a mobile day spa, a mobile salon that will cater to cancer patients."

"Wow," Mike said, "that's unique. Wow."

"A place that will be a wonderful and peaceful sanctuary for them. A palace on wheels, that will go to their curbside and pamper them with spa services and make them feel like a queen for a day."

"Yes," he said smiling, "that sounds amazing."

I told him we would offer these nurturing services to women with cancer: facial, manicure, pedicure, makeup and hair styling. I said that we could travel around Indiana doing these make-overs, making hundreds of women happy and changing their lives forever.

"YES!" he said again, louder. Mike was smiling more broadly with each idea, thinking of the positive impact we could make on all these people.

"And . . ."

"Yes?"

"AND . . ."

"YES?"

"And . . . all the services we would provide these women would be free," I said. "We will charge them *NOTHING!*"

I watched all the color slowly leave his face.

"Kim, how are we going to *pay* for this? How can we make a living for our family?" he asked.

"I don't know, I don't know how it's going to happen, but I know it's what we're supposed to do." We spent the next few miles in the car with me trying to convince him that this is what we were supposed to do. Mike was not buying into it, I could tell, but being the supportive husband that he is, he stopped at a bookstore in Kokomo and went inside the store to buy me three or four different books on "women and fund raising" and "women and nonprofits" and "grant writing for dummies"; anything he could find that would make this dream come true. He knew that once I set my mind to an idea there was no changing it.

I spent the next hour talking about this and how we would make this happen. Mike was not saying much and changing the subject every chance he got. About 30 miles from home our son woke up and we decided to take him into a play area so he could stretch his legs a little bit. As we were sitting there talking I looked at Mike and I said, "You know what. *This* is supposed to be called 'Hello Gorgeous!' because when these women feel the way that they do during their fight with cancer, that's how they deserve to be greeted. That's what they deserve to hear."

He still wouldn't talk to me about it and it took me several months to convince him. We held onto the salon for another year and then we sold it to concentrate our efforts fully on Hello Gorgeous! Since then Mike has worked six days a week, 12 hours a day at this for the last five years. I work three days a week as an independent stylist, in the salon we sold to pursue this dream, supporting our family as God unfolds this enormous and amazing journey out in front of us. Every woman we are able to help teaches us something. The hugs and tears of joy tell us we are on the right path, that we are making a difference. And Mike has told me that because of what he has seen with this project, and what he has learned from these Gorgeous Women, that even if he never gets paid to do this job, he will not quit.

So here are just a few of the amazing stories of the women we have had the distinct pleasure of serving through the Hello Gorgeous! Experience. Meeting them and listening to their stories has changed Mike and I and every member of our executive team forever. And we would like to share them with you. God Bless.

# LOVE

# love   (luhv)

*n.*

1. A deep, tender, ineffable feeling of affection and solitude for another, such as that arising from kinship or a sense of underlying oneness.
2. An expression of one's affection.
3. A strong predilection or enthusiasm.
4. Out of compassion; with no thought for a reward.

# One Definition of LOVE
# Our Gorgeous Women

THE FOLLOWING PAGES CONTAIN STORIES of some of the truly incredible women that it has been our pleasure to serve. Some of the stories here were written by Mike and I, some by their family or friends and others by the women themselves. I felt that I needed to tell these stories and share them with the world, because if I died tomorrow, all of these stories and their inspirations would never be told. They would die with me and I cannot have that happen.

So, this book is for all of our Gorgeous Women. It is also for you or a loved one who has been diagnosed, who are beginning your own journey with cancer. It is for the gallant cancer survivors that have gone through all these trials and the pain, and have come out on the other side of it a different person; not better, but maybe more thoughtful of life or more in love with it, no longer willing to waste it or let it pass them by. And it is for everyone who is not sick; who is well and living your fast and controlled life; unaware of how quickly things can change. Remember, according to the Beatles, that life is what happens while you are making other plans.

**"You will find as you look back upon your life
that the moments
when you have truly lived
are the moments when you
have done things in the spirit of Love."**

– *Henry Drummond*

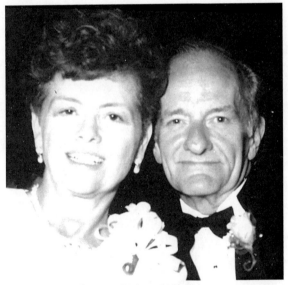

Hello
Gorgeous!

# Our First Gorgeous Woman
## (And We Did Not Know It)

Dr. Jeanine Becker and John Becker

WITHOUT REALIZING IT AT THE TIME, our very first Gorgeous! Woman was Mike's mother, Dr. Jeanine Becker.

I had the best mother-in-law on the face of the earth, even though she and I were not too sure of each other at the start. When I first started dating Mike, I referred to his parents as Mr. and Mrs. Becker. After a short period of time my future father-in-law said, "Kim, my name is John. Please call me John." But Mike's mom did not extend that same courtesy immediately. So for a long time Mike's parents were John and Mrs. Becker.

Mike's mom was a very intelligent and remarkable woman and was very into education. In 1992, when we met, Jeanine was a hospital administrator of 32 years. During the next 4 years, while working this high-stress position, she had also attended the University of Notre Dame and finished her Masters degree. And at the age of 58, she graduated from the University of Notre Dame with her Ph.D. The last year before her cancer she was invited to be an adjunct professor at the university she so dearly loved, teaching the young women of Notre Dame about the empowerment of women. I can think of no better teacher of this, but it did get in the way of our relationship a bit in the beginning.

I remember that after meeting me for the first time, Mike's mom questioned Mike candidly as to what degree I held. Mike explained to her that I was a hairdresser and that I did not have a college degree.

"Mike, I don't think that she is right for you," was her response. That *was* her response, I should say, until she experienced my *true* talent. That summer I was invited to attend a family vacation in Minnesota with Mike and his family. Now my mother-in-law was a classy woman, raised in that bygone age of the '50s and '60s when a woman went to the hairdresser once a week for a roller set and then wrapped her head in toilet paper each night to make it last until her next appointment! (Don't laugh too hard . . . your mother did it too!) So while we were on vacation I offered to do her hair for her.

"It is the least I can do," I said but it turned out to be the most perfect thing that could have happened. Again, Jeanine was a very classy lady and always wore heels, suits and scarves. But from the time I met her I felt that her hairstyle had dated her and, unbeknownst to her, I *could not wait* to get my hands on her hair!

That morning was the turning point in our relationship. I went from the "uneducated hairdresser that her son was dating" to a flat-out "Hair Wizard"!

Once I finished with her style she looked in the mirror and smiled. She walked over to her planner that she was *never* without and explained to me that, with my permission, she would like a standing 4:30 p.m. appointment every Friday and that she was going to write her current hairdresser and let him know that she now had a hairdresser in the family and that she was going to make a change. I WAS IN!

And on the day Mike and I got married, our Wedding Day, I did two heads of hair that morning: my mom and Mike's mom. I loved my mother-in-law. We had some great times and great laughs. Mike could always make her laugh. And for all her professional seriousness she had a child's loving, innocent heart and the kind of giggle that made you want to laugh out loud.

In the fall of 1996 Jeanine started not feeling well. She became a bit scatterbrained and forgetful, which was not like her at all. In early December Jeanine celebrated her 60th birthday. I was the party planner in the family and she insisted that I *not* throw her a party. She was very conscious of her age, as it pertained to the business world especially, and she did not want people knowing her true age. In mid-December Jeanine, Mike and I went shopping for Christmas gifts (it was our tradition) and she had what she thought was the flu. But the symptoms persisted and on December 21, 1996, we heard something we did not want to hear. Jeanine was diagnosed with a malignant brain tumor known as a

Glioblastoma. The doctor operated on Christmas Eve of that year and told us after the procedure that "it was exactly what he had expected." And what he had expected was not good.

I remember running out that very evening, Christmas Eve, speeding to the beauty supply store just as they were closing, pleading with them to let us in so that Mike and I could purchase a couple of terrycloth turbans to cover Jeanine's shaved head. I knew nothing about caring for a cancer victim as a cosmetologist at that time and I felt a little ashamed that I did not know exactly what to do for her. But I was going to work hard to do what I could.

I will never forget walking into Jeanine's hospital room Christmas Eve night and in my total amazement, hours after brain surgery, she was sitting up in bed drinking cappuccino, talking and smiling, and laughing. She truly was an amazing woman. (And I never realized how much Mike and his mom looked alike, until I saw them both with no hair!)

Upon her release from the hospital they administered six weeks of radiation, five days a week, and then chemotherapy. I put my hairdressing skills into action and went to work on arranging for Jeanine to get a wig and a headband with bangs that could be worn with her terrycloth turbans.

She always loved having her nails done. So we kept her Friday standing appointments at 4:30 for, if nothing else, to wash and massage her scalp for her (which she loved), to manicure her nails for her, and to spend precious time with someone I loved.

One Friday I had noticed that the hair on her head had started growing back in and she and I were both very excited. It was a beautiful salt and pepper color coming back in and we even had enough of it to trim. Unfortunately, that hair did not last. During one of her next Friday appointments, as

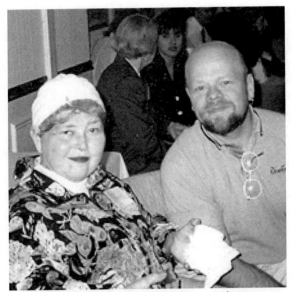

Michael and Our Jeanine at Tribute to Women Gathering

I was shampooing this gorgeous hair of hers, it began falling out in my hands. The strainer in the sink now held the beautiful salt-and-pepper-colored hair that once sat on the head of my beautiful mother-in-law. That was a tough day for me, for both of us. I now had to tell Jeanine that we would have to wait a while longer for her own hair to grow back in. We both had a good laugh and a good cry at the shampoo bowl that Friday. But we went through it together.

As time went on Jeanine started to get progressively worse. I would ask God on a regular basis, "WHY?" The very things that she had worked *so hard for* her entire life—her knowledge, her education, her mind—were the very things that the cancer was greedily taking from her. The doctors had given her six months. She lasted only 14 weeks.

Jeanine died on April 12, 1997. She was at home and it was a Saturday night. My father-in-law, John, is a caring and loving man and made sure that she would die at home without pain, whatever the cost. Mike and I, his dad John, and Mike's sister Maria were playing a board game at the kitchen table, adjacent to the room where Jeanine lay in her hospital bed. She was on morphine to control the pain. Well, the game we were playing got a bit competitive and we were all taunting each other and laughing honestly and fully, like Jeanine used to do. We knew she could hear us through the pain, through the unconsciousness. And I think she knew we were all there for her, close, sending her our love. It was a good moment in a tragic situation.

That was when it happened. Her pain was gone, but so was our Jeanine.

It was a very peaceful passing and I am honored to have been there. Jeanine had started her career as a nurse and had three very close nursing friends from all those years ago. They had all met in nursing school 40 years before, as teenagers, worked together during their careers at the hospital and had made a pact at some point that each of them would be there for the others when their time came to die. Sylvia, Phyllis and Joanne were called before anyone else, so that their pact could be kept. They came and said their goodbyes, cleaned her up to keep her dignity for her, and knew in their hearts that nothing would ever be the same again.

My in-laws had always talked about getting a Prevost RV and traveling the country so that Jeanine could speak on the empowerment of women and my father-in-law, a 32-year firefighter, would drive the bus. I feel in some way that we are carrying on that aspiration for her with Hello Gorgeous! And every time we speak publicly, I know that she is giggling like the young girl at heart that she was.

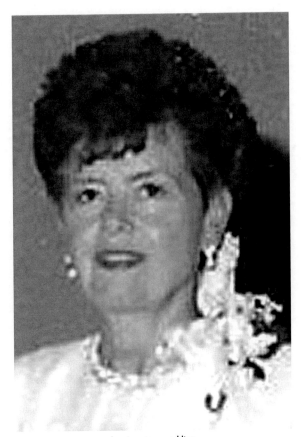

Jeanine at our wedding

Jeanine was our first Gorgeous! Woman and we didn't even know it. We had no idea at that time what God had in store for us and how our experience with Jeanine would help us empower women all over the world.

Thanks, Mom. Love you and I miss you.

# Tena

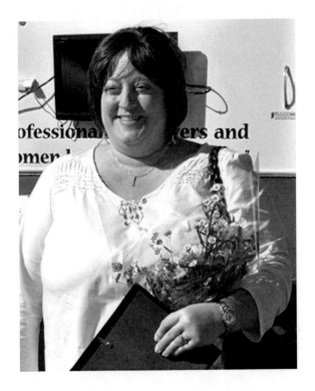

## Battle Wounds

# Hello Gorgeous!

TENA WAS OUR FIRST GORGEOUS WOMAN *ever* done in the mobile DaySpa. And we certainly picked the right lady! I asked her to write her story and we are so glad she did:

> Sadly, we all know someone—a mother, a sister, a friend, a neighbor—who has faced or is facing breast cancer. In November of 2009 I felt a lump in my breast that had not been there the night before. Yes, I did daily exams, not monthly. My sister was diagnosed with breast cancer 16 years ago at the age of 35, so it was pounded into our heads to do self-checks. Thank God I did. I saw my family doctor the next day, had a mammogram the day after that and a biopsy the following week. What sticks in my mind, from that time, was the radiologist doctor telling me after my mammogram that he was 99.9% sure it was not cancerous and, if it were not for my sister previously having cancer, he would not do the biopsy but make me wait 3-6 months and come back in for another mammogram. But, since there was a history of cancer with an immediate family member, he was going to leave the decision up to me.
>
> I took the option of the biopsy. I wasn't taking

> *Out of suffering have emerged the strongest souls; the most massive characters are seared with scars.*
> – Edwin H. Chapin

31

a chance and I could not live with seeing and feeling that lump for the next 3-6 months! I had the biopsy done the following Thursday. On Monday, I received a call from my family doctor telling me that I needed to see a surgeon "sooner rather than later" and that was the start of my journey to where I am today. I had a lumpectomy and 3 lymph nodes removed just before Christmas along with a port being put in for chemo. The scars at first reminded me of the cancer and I associated them with negative feelings, but since then, I have changed that and they have become my battle wounds—badges of honor to show that I am a survivor. I'm very proud of my scars; they remind me not of cancer, but that I BEAT cancer. Not long after Christmas I started my six rounds of chemo. Just after my second round of chemo I started losing my hair. I remember calling my husband crying and telling him that it was time to see Lori (one of my best friends as well as my hairstylist) and have her shave my head. I made the appointment and we headed down that night. It

> *Some people care
> too much,
> I think it's called love.*
> *– Winnie the Pooh*

was an emotional night as my best friend shaved not only my head, but my husband's too. We were in this together. I did not look at myself until we got home. To make me laugh, my daughters came up with reasons why it would be great to have no hair. I could get ready in the morning faster, did not have to buy shampoo or conditioner and the best one was that I would not have a bad hair day.

In March of 2010, my husband told me we had to go to TGI Friday's because his company was celebrating a job that they had gotten. I thought it was odd that he asked if I was going to wear my wig...well, duh, we are going out and I need to be dressed up. I would soon find out why he was worried that I would not wear the wig. We arrived and sat in the bar and I kept looking at my watch and asking, "Where is everyone? Are they blowing us off?" The next thing I knew someone walked in and asked if Tena was here. I turned around and there was Kim from Hello Gorgeous! I was so surprised! Lori and my husband had conspired together and nominated me for a makeover. What I also didn't know was that a co-worker had nominated me as well. They took me to the Hello Gorgeous! mobile DaySpa, in the restaurant parking lot, and started my makeover. I felt like a princess. My daughters both were there as well as my whole family. I could not believe everyone had kept this so quiet. The makeover started and I received a manicure and pedicure which I had never had before . . . can I just say I LOVED IT! I received a massage and a facial and then was taken to the back of the mobile spa for my new hairstyle. They had three wigs (plus the one that I had already). One was similar to how my hair was before and another was totally different. It had blond on the top with brown underneath and was short. I picked the blond one, which shocked Lori.

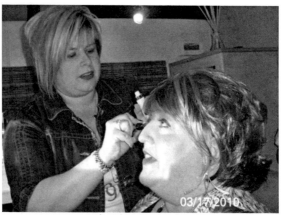
Trish applying Tena's makeup

I would have never tried that color or style, but it made me feel good and I figured if I were going to lose my hair, I was going to have some fun with it. I finished my makeover with a new outfit and felt like a million dollars. I could not stop smiling.

When I walked out of the mobile spa and saw my husband, all I wanted to do was run to him and give him a big hug! I wish every woman going through cancer could experience this feeling. Going through surgery and chemo, along with feeling like crap all of the time, is bad enough but then to lose your hair. Nothing can prepare you for that. No matter how much you think it will not bother you, until you are faced with the reality that your hair is gone, you cannot say how you will react. It might sound vain, but society identifies us by our looks and your hair is a big part of you. So this makeover was not just a "make you feel good for a day" makeover. A few days after my makeover, I was going through the Starbucks drive-thru and the cashier at the window told me how much she loved my hair. I was so shocked! Since you know you are wearing a wig, you assume everyone else can tell. You are very self-conscious about it. But this comment made my day! It was not long after that that I was at the Dollar Tree store and the cashier there also told me how much she loved the cut and color of my hair. I just smiled and thanked her. Those two comments from strangers remind me how much of an impact our words have on others. A kind word to someone can change their whole day. You cannot always tell what kind of hell someone else is going through. We are always so quick to judge others. A kind word or just a smile is all it takes and that's what Hello Gorgeous! did for me. For a few hours, I was able to forget that I had cancer; forget that I had doctor's appointments, hospital bills, mom duties and everyday things to do. This time was just for me. My world stopped for just a little while. It was what I needed. No matter how down you are, these women can pick you up and make you feel so special. They are an amazing team and so blessed to be able to do this work. I cannot imagine being able to make someone who is at one of the lowest points of their life feel beautiful and special.

I finished chemo on April 13 and I was off to "Camp Nukemboobie" as I called it, to start my 27 rounds of radiation treatments. The beginning of radiation went fine. No burns. I kept wondering if I was going to luck out and not have any burning or if it was going to sneak up on me. It snuck up. The burns were manageable, but they were painful.

The physician's assistant at the oncologists' office had told me about using a cabbage leaf on the burns. I decided to try it since the lotion they were giving me would come off on my clothing, so it really did not help to even put it on. Since I could not wear a Band-Aid, as I am allergic to the glue and it would only aggravate the burn along with the area around the burn (tried it once and it tore off some of my skin), I used a panty-liner, it too just soaked up the lotion, but worked wonderfully when I had to have a biopsy done later. I have to say, the cabbage worked amazingly! It cooled the burn and kept a barrier between my clothes and skin. Sad that a $0.59 head of cabbage worked better than the $300 tube of medicine they gave me. On my final radiation day, I went and had two tattoos done. One on my wrist to always remind me how far I have come and the other is a red rose with the breast cancer ribbon around it and the date of my last treatment under it.

During the time of my journey, I met some amazing people. On my first day of chemo I sat next to a gentleman who was given six months to live. It was two years ago when he was first told that. When I went for my six-month check-up, guess who was there? This man had the most positive attitude on life and he is the reason my husband and I laughed throughout the course of my treatment. If I would have sat around being nervous about it, then I would have missed everything else. Yes, you have to give yourself time to grieve but if you allow it to consume your life, the grief will *become* your life.

I do not think cancer took anything away from me. If anything, it gave to me:

- Confidence that I am a strong woman.
- A stronger relationship with my husband.
- A voice, not only to stand my ground with a doctor because of a G.U.T. instinct (God's Ultimate Thought), but to also tell other women to do self-exams, no matter your age.
- A reminder to enjoy every day that you are given.

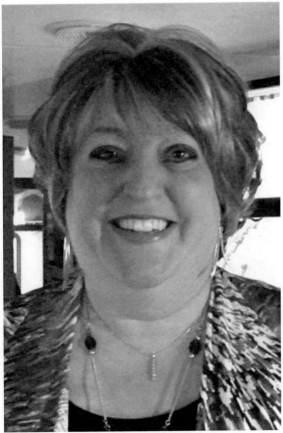

Tena after her makeover

- Opportunities to meet wonderful people that are out there helping other cancer patients become survivors.
- And, the "funniest" thing that cancer gave me was the opportunity to become a blond with short, spiky hair.

# Tena's Update

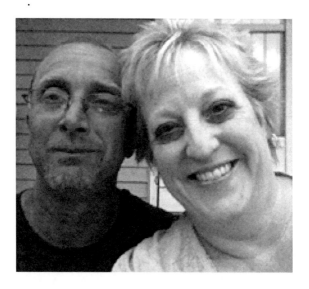

Today, I am cancer free. I am proud to say that I am a breast cancer survivor.

# Cheryl

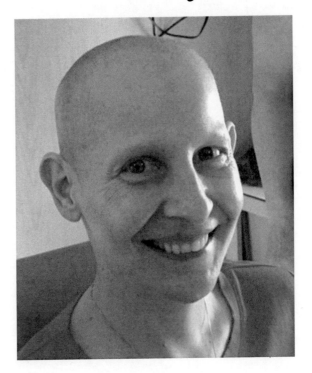

"Wow, I don't look sick."

# Hello Gorgeous!

CHERYL WAS THE FIRST LADY for whom we received two nominations, from two different people, who did not know each other. We knew that this was someone we were supposed to help. Here is the nomination received in October of 2009. Her friend Rhonda wrote:

*"My friend Cheryl has been living and dealing with this disease for eight years now. Throughout it all she has remained determined to fight as long and as hard as possible despite going through so many treatments and side-effects, complications and challenges along the way.*

*Along the way she still managed to care for several older and ailing relatives, as well as her two girls and husband as best she could. Cheryl also managed to keep an adventurous spirit throughout the journey, taking vacations to places she'd always wanted to go, when most in her condition would be leery or afraid to do so. This is just another testament to her perseverance, in my opinion. She seems to put many persons' needs ahead of her own, always making sure to remember a special event or date or even some little things to make it special. I hope she continues to fight this battle and hope this gift will make her feel as loved and appreciated as the friend she has always been. Her chemo treatments are now done and she has reached all the possibilities for*

41

*any more effectiveness and time is of the essence. I would love the possibility of a beauty day in a private-salon setting with a couple of the other girls to get her any type of joy possible. Thank you so much and God bless."*

Cheryl's cancer started out as cervical cancer. Four years into her remission the cervical cancer had metastasized to her lung and liver. Unbelievably, Cheryl received her 194th chemotherapy treatment on October of 2009. It was at this point that the doctors decided there was no more they could do for her.

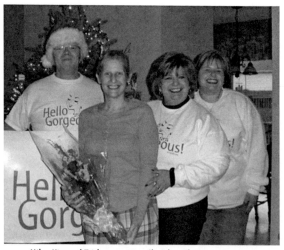

Mike, Kim and Trisha surprising Cheryl on Christmas morning

One of our favorite moments with Hello Gorgeous! was when we surprised Cheryl, at her home, on Christmas Day that year. We showed up that morning at her house, unannounced, and presented her with candy and flowers and a big "Hello Gorgeous!" We presented her with a certificate and told her that, when she was ready and feeling up to it, she could call and we would come out with the mobile

DaySpa and pamper her and give her a day of beauty. That was in December of 2009. In April of 2010 we got a phone call from her friend. She said that they were ready for the mobile unit: it was getting harder for Cheryl to breathe and to get around but she was very excited for the visit. And they wanted to have this done before Cheryl became too sick to enjoy it.

It was a beautiful April day when we rolled the red carpet out on her lawn and escorted her onto the DaySpa. To this day Cheryl is one of the most resilient and joyous women I have ever met. Knowing her disease, and the pain she must have been in, she was all smiles and eagerness. It was as if looking forward to this day allowed her to overcome it. So we all made the most of it.

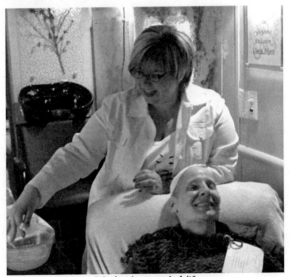

"The facial was wonderful!"

Cheryl had a relaxing facial, a pedicure and a manicure. She was a hairdresser by trade, used to giving beauty treatments to other people, so she especially enjoyed having them done on herself. We did her makeup for her and then approached her hairstyle. Her hair was very short and fuzzy. She didn't like wigs very much so she rarely wore them, even through all her years of chemotherapy. But we thought that we had the *perfect* wig for her; it was a headband with hair attached, no bang, and it was very low maintenance. She agreed to try it so we trimmed the wig up a bit and put it on. She looked amazing! And what Cheryl said next, when we turned her toward the mirror, is one of those moments I will remember forever.

"Oh my gosh, I don't look sick!"

How amazing is *that* for someone to say after 200 chemotherapy treatments! And she just kept smiling that radiant smile of hers. But we were not done yet. We arranged for Cheryl and her two girlfriends to go to lunch at a local restaurant (familiar with Hello Gorgeous! and its mission) after our visit with her. Trisha, our Creative Director, called the restaurant to explain what was going on and described the three women who would be coming to their restaurant that afternoon. It was an elegant establishment and Cheryl loved the atmosphere as soon as she walked in; but when the manager, the hostess and their waiter all met them at the door with "Hello Gorgeous!" (*unprompted* by us), she was overwhelmed. It was a great day and Cheryl was an amazing woman. It was a wonderful experience spending time with her.

# Cheryl's Update

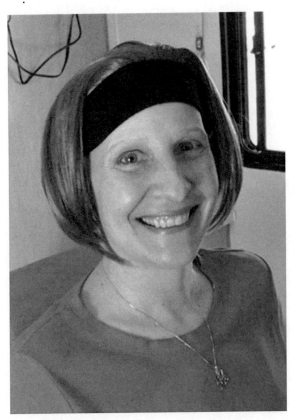

In October 2010, Cheryl lost her battle with cancer. But she fought with a grace and resilience that continues to inspire those who knew her. Her girlfriends that had nominated her for our visit called me and told me that it was a very peaceful ending. And when I went to the funeral home to show my respect, to my tearful amazement, the pictures of that sparkling day that Cheryl spent with us were included in the other photographs that had been chosen to represent Cheryl's life on this earth. There was no doubt in my mind that we had made a difference for Cheryl and her family. And every time I see her pictures with us that day, I am reminded of the power that a single act of kindness can wield in someone else's life, as well as your own.

# Melissa

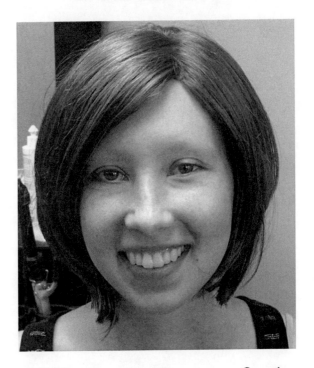

"They made me feel
beautiful
when I felt so ugly."

# Hello Gorgeous!

MELISSA IS A VERY YOUNG AND VIVACIOUS 24-year-old. She was diagnosed with Ewing Sarcoma and it was found in her uterus. Her friend Laura nominated her and wrote:

*"I cannot put into words how hard Melissa's struggle has been for her and [her husband] Jeff. They were married for a little over a year and a half before she was diagnosed with a small lump in her uterus. Just before Melissa's surgery, Jeff was laid off from his job as a construction worker. With both of them unable to work there were several months when only the Lord's provision and strength got them through it all. But they always remained positive. It's hard enough for newlyweds to deal with the cancer, but now Melissa is struggling with how she looks as well. She has been so strong and has been through so many trials in the past seven months. We cannot take the cancer from her, but we can help her take her appearance off of her mind. I have tried to help her with makeup and such things, but my knowledge of it is limited. Please consider Melissa as a deserving candidate for your services and thank you for all that you do for women like her."*

It was in January 2009 that she was diagnosed. Our visit with her was in August. We did not have the mobile day spa yet so we were doing the services in our former salon. We had sold it three years before, to focus all of our efforts on

Hello Gorgeous!, but I [Kim] continued to work there to support our family financially, as I still do. To get Melissa to the salon, her friend Laura told her that she (Laura) had won a manicure by winning a sales contest that they had held at their workplace, and hoped that Melissa would come along with her for the experience. After reading this nomination I could not even imagine how it would feel to be that young, to be a newlywed and to deal with those issues. But her faith in the Lord is strong and she will get through this. What an amazing, strong-spirited, young woman. Here is her story in her own words:

> I was 23 when I woke up from surgery. I had gone in for a routine surgery to have a fibroid tumor removed; I woke up to my doctor telling me that I had cancer and that he had to perform a hysterectomy (removal of the uterus). Within about a ten-second time frame, I found out I was an infertile cancer patient. I never thought I would be there.
>
> I don't remember much about the time I spent waiting to start chemo. It was a whirlwind of tests, doctor appointments, and more tests. There were scans, blood work, biopsies, EKG's, and more to diagnose what type of cancer I had and to get me ready for the treatment ahead. For me, this was the part of my treatment that was the hardest. All I could do was wait to find out if I was going to live or die. I had never felt so scared, desperate, abandoned, and forgotten. I hated going to see the oncologists. I hated the word oncology and I hated the word cancer. I was angry. I felt like God forgot to watch over me and protect me. Oops, Melissa has cancer.
>
> In the beginning, the emotions and weight of

the situation were simply just too much for me to handle. Between my tests and doctor appointments, the only energy I could muster was to get up in the mornings, go lie on the couch, and pretend to sleep. I could only pretend. I couldn't sleep. I could only pray, and I prayed constantly. I prayed the same prayers over and over again all day long. I prayed for healing, and I prayed Bible verses that offered encouragement. I didn't know what else to do. I just wanted to die. I didn't want to go through what I knew was ahead.

One of the scariest moments of my life was early after my diagnosis. We had received a diagnosis of Ewing Sarcoma of the uterus (this is a rare pediatric cancer that can be found in young adults). If the cancer had not spread I had a very good prognosis; they thought I would be cured. If the cancer had spread, I was given a 20% chance of survival.

I was lying in my hospital bed at the University of Chicago Children's hospital and had just come back from surgery to have my medication port placed. I would be receiving chemo through this port. Since I was being treated by pediatricians, I was treated as a pediatric patient. Adults are usually awake when they have a bone marrow biopsy. They had taken my bone marrow while I was asleep in surgery, so I did not have to be awake for this painful test. This test was the last place they were looking to see if they could see if the cancer had spread. The doctor walked into my room at 4:25 on a Friday afternoon to check on me and see how I was doing, Five minutes before, the lab where my bone marrow was being tested closed. The first thing out of my mouth was to ask what the results were. She didn't have the results yet, so she stepped out to make the call to the lab. In those moments as I lay there waiting for her to return, I remember feeling my heart pound like I had never felt it pound before. This was the moment I was going to learn if I had a greater chance to live, or a greater chance to die. These test results were about to shed some light on how hard my fight was going to be. The doctor then walked back into the room and gave me the news. It had not spread!

I then started chemo. I received five different chemo drugs to make sure there were no microscopic cancer cells left in my body. I had three chemo drugs the first week and then had a week to recover. Then I had two chemo drugs over a week and another week to recover. On my weeks I had off from treatment I had to come into the office every other day to have blood work since the chemo was so hard on my body. My oncologist's office was my second home. I did this regimen for eight long months before having six weeks of radiation that concluded my cancer treatment.

It was a long, dark year with no end in sight. I felt old and sick, I hurt everywhere, and I had lost all of my hair. I even lost my nose hair. I was pale and sickly looking. I tried to cover up the physical evidence of going through chemo, but I could tell I was not fooling anyone when I would go out in public. There was no ignoring the stares. It felt like treatment would never end. All I wanted to do was finish treatment, move on with my life, and start a family.

But every once in a while, when you are going through something that is harder than comprehension, God sends some hope, a little glimmer of light leading you to the end of the tunnel. This hope seems to come when you least expect. He gives just a little boost to cheer you on, encourage, and keep you pushing to the finish line. I was just past the half-way point of my treatment when a friend of mine told me that she had won a free mani/pedi for herself and a friend. She asked if I wanted to go with her and I gladly accepted.

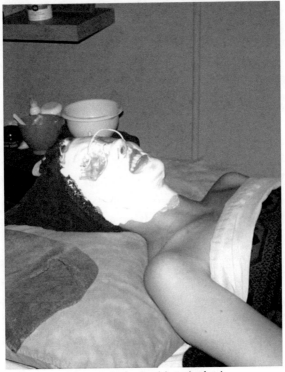

Melissa completely relaxed during her facial.

We walked into the salon and I was greeted with flowers, gifts, and "Hello Gorgeous!" It was the warmest welcome I had ever received. I was just about to explain to these people that it was my friend that had won the contest, when they explained what was really going on. They must have read the confusion on my face! I was in disbelief. They pampered me from head to toe that day. They made me feel beautiful when I felt so ugly. I had a facial and a massage. They painted my fingers and my toes; they did my make up and taught me how to draw eyebrows. I felt like a girl again. They put my wig on me and I looked in the mirror. I didn't feel ugly, and I didn't feel like a freak anymore. I actually felt pretty. I felt like I could walk outside and not be afraid of people staring. I could hold my head up in confidence again. They had given me a day away from cancer. Hello Gorgeous! helped me persevere.

Hello Gorgeous! is made up of some of the biggest-hearted, genuine people you can ever meet. They give because they love so much. Even though I understand what it's like to go through something very hard, sometimes I forget too quickly what it might mean to someone else if I were to share my story and talk with them. I am a nurse and I meet a lot of cancer patients. Because of the love Hello Gorgeous! gave to me, it reminds me to always share my story with others fighting cancer. Sometimes they aren't at a place in their experience where they are ready to take in what I have to say. Sometimes they are, and when they are, I can see it in their eyes. I can see the hope. When I see the hope in their eyes, it makes my experience mean so much more. Hope is everything. Hoping in something more than yourself keeps you going, gives you life. God used Hello Gorgeous! in my life to give me hope, and I pray that He uses my experience to give hope to others.

Thank you for reading my story. Thank you, Hello Gorgeous! for being part of something bigger than yourself and for letting me share my story. Mostly, thank you, God, for giving hope.

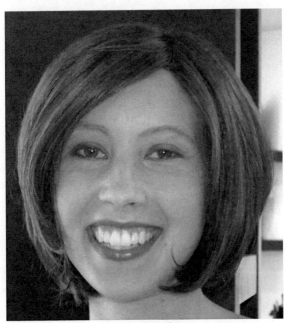

Melissa after her makeover

## Melissa's Update

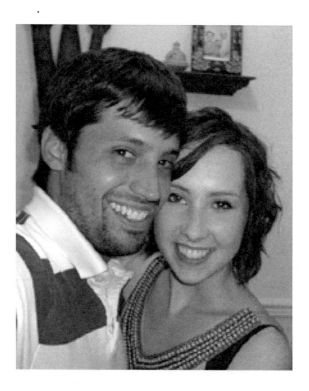

Right now I'm having scans every six months. I will be two years out from treatment on Christmas Eve 2011. I have not had a doctor tell me I am cured or in remission, so I have just decided to start over and I am taking what I have learned along the way with me.

# Linda

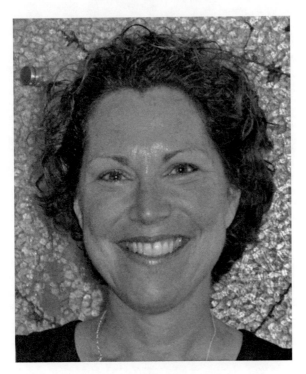

## "You Must Have the Wrong Person!"

Hello Gorgeous!

LINDA IS FROM CARMEL, INDIANA. Linda's nomination came to us through an organization called IWIN (Indiana Women In Need). We had the great pleasure of meeting her on our six-week tour last summer. When I received the nomination, it stated:

> Linda had come to the IWIN foundation in 2007 after being diagnosed with breast cancer. The foundation provided meals, massage therapy and housekeeping for her and her family while she was going through treatment. At the time Linda had twin two-year-old boys. Since then she has had a re-occurrence of her cancer, she continues to keep up with twin sons, and has become separated from her husband. We feel she is deserving of the Hello Gorgeous! Experience after all that she has been through. Linda was diagnosed with cancer in August of 2007 and then was re-diagnosed in November of 2008.

We found out that Linda's mom had gone through breast cancer as well. When we met Linda she was inside the Paradise Café at Hamilton Town Center in Noblesville, Indiana. We had arranged for a camera crew from Channel 6 in Indianapolis to join us. Here is Linda's visit, in her own words:

> I don't think I've ever had a bigger smile on my face than I did on June 27, 2010. On that day, I thought I was out having an ordinary lunch

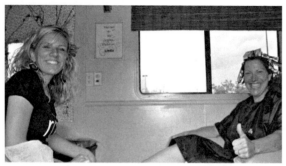

Darci from Rain Salon performing a pedicure on Linda

with my mom and sister, but it turned out to be anything but ordinary. Upon arriving at the restaurant, the Hello Gorgeous! team jumped into action. They swarmed me at the table and informed me that I had been chosen to receive a day of pampering.

"You must have the wrong person," I thought. It didn't seem real. Was someone playing a joke on me? Where were the hidden cameras?

The Hello Gorgeous! team came prepared to make this a day one that I would always remember; complete with a certificate, flowers and a makeover including hair, nails, facial, makeup and clothes. Cameras were rolling and I was speechless. Me? What did I do to deserve this? Who would have nominated me for such an awesome experience? Let me start from the beginning:

My husband and I married in April 2003. We were blessed with twin boys born January 2006. Along with my two step kids, we now had four children. An instant large "blended" family brought many challenges, some too much to handle at the time. My husband and I separated in July 2006, all the while keeping in touch and helping take care of the twins. Time passed, and in September 2007, I found a lump in my right breast. A mammogram could not detect the lump, but did find calcifications, which ended up testing positive for cancer. After two surgeries, I was treated with six-and-a-half weeks of radiation. During this time, family, friends and neighbors helped care for the twins, prepared meals and cleaned my home. I couldn't have done it without them. After my next mammogram in April, it appeared this treatment worked. I was cancer free, or so I thought.

Six months later, in October 2008, during a follow-up mammogram, my life was about to change in a major way. The results showed new cancer cells in the same breast. I could not believe what I was hearing. No way! How could this be happening? Again! How could I NOT beat the odds! This time I was in for a much more radical treatment. A bilateral mastectomy was scheduled for January 30, 2009, the day before my twins' third birthday. I'm a stay-at-home mom and my husband and I were still separated. How was I going to do this? Well, with a lot of faith and a lot of help, I made it through the eleven-hour surgery and eight weeks of recovery.

My last check-up was in January 2011, and this time I AM cancer free! Also in January, my husband and I reconciled. We just recently moved into a new house, all six of us. The twins started kindergarten, my stepson is a senior in high school and my stepdaughter is a junior in college. Life is good. I have God to thank for that and the many people who stood by me and prayed their hearts out.

\* \* \* \* \*

Now back to June 27, 2010. I soon realized this was not a joke, but a reality. This was happening to me! I was nominated by a friend and Hello Gorgeous! picked me to receive this special day of beauty. I felt like a movie star! I was whisked over to the Hello Gorgeous! DaySpa and the pampering started. Everyone was fussing over ME. When has THAT ever happened? I received a haircut and color, manicure, pedicure, facial, makeup and a smashing new outfit. To top it all off, they informed me I would "reveal the new me" in front of a crowd of friends and family. Oh, what a blast that was. I was introduced as the new "hot mama." Everyone was so surprised and so glad to see me so happy. Can't wipe that smile off of my face! I smile every time I think about it.

You know, life throws a lot of curve balls at you which you have no control over. The key is to

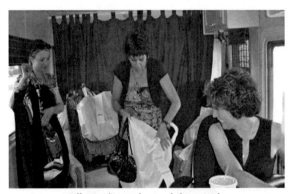

Tiffany and Leeca showing clothes to Linda

not let them get you down. Oh, I'm not saying it's easy to stay chipper all the time. It's hard when you don't feel well and you have to take care of small children too. Just know that having a strong will and a strong faith will get you through just about anything. And just know that there are people out there who care and who will help in ways unimaginable. Just like Hello Gorgeous! did for me. Thank you, Hello Gorgeous!, and thanks to everyone who helped me throw those curve balls back!

Linda is an amazing individual. Her two sons are the light of her life and I believe that is what kept her going. Her smile never quit that day we were with her. It lit up the room. When we got her all done she had no idea we were going to have the after-party. When we walked into the room, I had everybody greet her with a big "Hello Gorgeous!" As soon as she walked in, her two boys found her and they ran into her open arms. You could certainly tell that they were her inspiration to keep going every day.

And, in the same way, her story keeps us going every day as well.

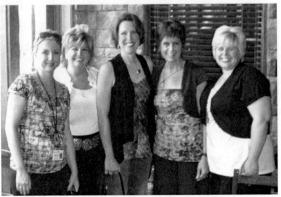

Tiffany, Kim, our Gorgeous Woman Linda, Leeca and Trisha at the Reveal

## Linda's Update

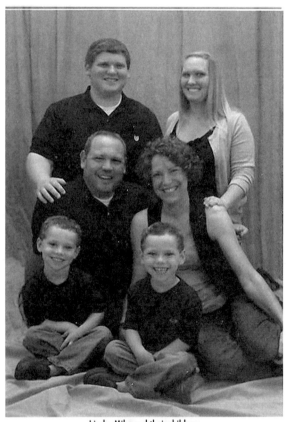

Linda, Mike and their children

Linda is now in remission. She still has that dazzling smile and has reconciled with her husband, Mike. The children are all well and the twins have started kindergarten.

# Karen

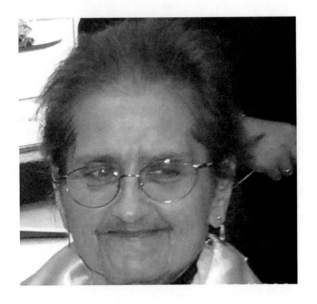

"Humming the theme to
'Miss America'"

## Hello Gorgeous!

WE WERE ABLE TO MEET KAREN on January 26, 2009, three days after her birthday. Her daughter Kelly wrote us and told us a little about Karen and why her mom deserved a day of beauty:

> "My name is Kelly and my mom's name is Karen. Diagnosed with leiomyosarcoma in November 2004 she went through chemotherapy and radiation. She lost all of her hair and fingernails, and was hospitalized for five week due to her organs failing. Her husband passed away in October 2005 of lung cancer. She has had a long hard battle with this. She is also in a wheelchair due to an amputated leg 12 years ago. I am an only child and a lot rests on my shoulders. I think my mom deserves to be pampered for a few hours and get some of her self-esteem back. She is currently in Goshen hospital they had to put in a shunt to help circulate the fluid in her body. Her tumor is currently lying in an artery and is causing it not to function properly. I really hope that you can do this for my mom. She has helped so many people in so many ways during her life and now she can use a little help herself."

The day we met Karen, she had finished all her treatments and there was nothing more that the doctors could do for her, due to the location of her tumor. She came to the salon to have her pampering done—her day of beauty—because we did not have the mobile day spa at the time. It was a very snowy January day. Kelly had needed the help of three other people to pull her mom through the deep snow and into the salon in her wheelchair. Mike, Trisha and I surprised Karen with a *"Hello Gorgeous!"* in addition to a surprise of flowers and candy and told her she had been nominated for a day of beauty and that she had been chosen to receive several spa services that day. Kelly explained to us that Karen was having a lot of pain that day and that she may not be up to all of the things we had planned. We assured Kelly that that was fine and that we would do whatever her mother felt comfortable doing.

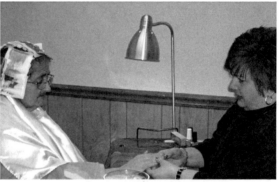
Karen enjoying her manicure

Her facial was first, then a manicure. We even did a pedicure on her single foot and Karen thought that was great. After each service, Karen talked a little more, sat a little higher in her wheelchair and smiled more often. She had hair, so we were able to highlight and cut it. We did some facial waxing on her and some makeup. And when we had finished, the transformation was absolutely amazing, inside and out.

There was a hardware store right next to the salon and men of all ages would walk right past the plate-glass window all day long. At one point that afternoon Karen looked out the

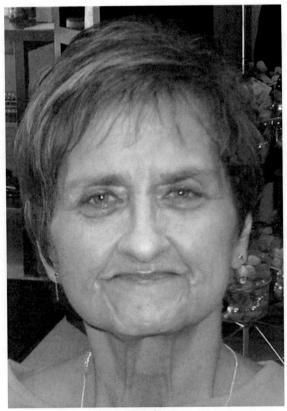

Karen after

window and said: "Mike, go grab one of those men for me and bring him back here! Let's find out if they're single."

This was certainly a far cry from the Karen who came into the salon too pained, depressed and beaten down to even speak.

Two days after Karen's visit we got this e-mail from her daughter, it said:

> "Hi ladies, this is Kelly. I just wanted to let you know that during our experience on Monday my mom had a wonderful time. From the time we arrived there to the time we walked out the door,

you made her feel like she was on top of the world. You are so thoughtful and caring to do things like this for women: to make them feel beautiful again after going through such an ugly disease. As we left the makeover, my mom was humming the theme to 'Miss America.' It was good to see her happy and her old self again. You treated her like a special person, not just a customer and, when you cried when we were leaving, that showed us exactly what kind of people you really are. You are amazing and I wish that there were more people like you in the world. It would be a much better place. I will keep in touch. Thank you so much for making my mom happy for a day. I wish that we could have it in our lives every day.

Sincerely and with much thanks and love,

Karen and Kelly"

# Karen's Update

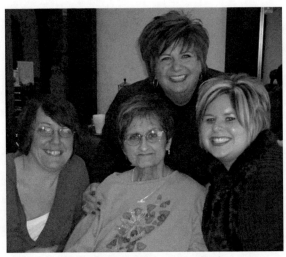

Karen's daughter Kelly, Karen, Kim and Trisha

That summer in June, Karen lost her battle with cancer and Kelly called to let us know that she had passed. When we went to the funeral home to and were standing in line waiting to pay our respects, we noticed there was a video playing of all Karen's life pictures—from the time she was a young child until the time she had passed. As we stood there and watched the video, the pictures of her day with us in the salon were on that video. I thought to myself, what an amazing gift—we had spent only four hours with this wonderful individual and yet we made the story of her life! She has forever changed ours and you begin to realize exactly how precious life is and what an amazing gift we all have to share. Karen *was* "Miss America" in our book.

# Heather

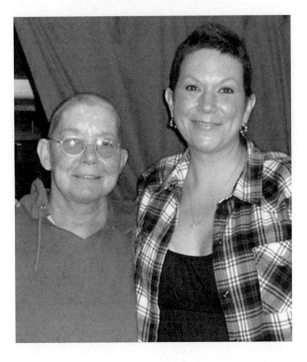

## "I Made Peace with My Body"

# Hello Gorgeous!

I WAS FORTUNATE THAT HEATHER volunteered to tell her own story and we are all fortunate that she is a very good story-teller. Heather's story is a prime example of how fast cancer can happen and how it can consume your life.

In June of 2011, June 16 to be exact, I was diag-nosed with breast cancer. I was 34 years old, just starting to get back into shape after having my youngest daughter Lia a year-and-a-half earlier, and a stay-at-home mom to both Lia and my older daughter, Camryn, who is 10. I was also a wife and homemaker, cook and chauffeur, and everything else that comes along with being a wife (in a young family with children) with a self-employed husband. And it was while enjoying some (very rare, I might add) "alone time" with my husband that I first noticed the lump under my right breast. It felt like a smallish egg under my skin. I did not know how in the WORLD I hadn't noticed it before. I showed the area to Tim, and although he was very calm and reassuring, he did agree that I should see my doctor as soon as possible, which I did.

To my unpleasant surprise, I was asked a barrage of questions regarding my family history, the location and shape of the lump, if I had any pain or nipple discharge, and I got in within two days of making my call. Upon examination, my doctor was quite certain that it was a fibrous cyst (I had very dense, very big, fibrous (a.k.a. lumpy) breasts). It felt round and smooth and it didn't hurt. I had no family history of breast cancer, no "dimpling" of the skin on my breast, no redness or tenderness, and I was in my 30s. I had nothing to worry about. He wanted me to come back in three weeks (later in my menstrual cycle) to see if it changed in size due to my hormones. I came back and everything seemed fine. We were going to "wait and see."

In the meantime, it became my new distraction. I was always feeling, poking and prodding it. I still felt quite uneasy about it. By this time our tenth wedding anniversary was coming up, and we had booked a week-long trip to Negril, Jamaica, at a very secluded resort in a lush tropical setting. Still, the lump bothered me. It bothered *me* enough that it bothered my husband, if that makes any sense. I had my annual exam coming up with my gynecologist, so I waited until after our vacation to make my appointment. But after we got back, things moved very quickly.

I had my annual pap exam and told my gynecologist about the lump. He checked it out and pretty much agreed with what my family doctor had said—it's round, smooth, painless, you're in your 30s with no family history. "This isn't anything that's going to be dangerous to you," he told me, "but let's get this checked out because something that is palpable like this will need to be drained if it's a cyst or you're going to want it removed if its fibrous." Then he ordered a mammogram for me. So I went in for my first mammogram at age 34, a full 6 years before the "official recommended age." It wasn't painful or uncomfortable like I had imagined, and the tech and I were talking about our children; how we had both breastfed and how that was supposed to offer some protection against breast cancer. She left to have the doctor look at the films and came back to say that she needed more images. She left again, came back and again needed *more* images. The third time that she came in, she said that the radiologist wanted me to have an ultrasound on my breast.

Right now . . . as in pushing back a pregnant woman's ultrasound appointment to do mine.

As I was lying in the ultrasound room, I was talking to the tech in there about my kids, doing anything to keep calm. My husband was with me, as were our daughters. When the technician went to get the radiologist to look at the images, I had my eldest daughter, Camryn, go out and push her little sister around the halls in her stroller. I am so glad I did that. The radiologist said that although my lump felt round and smooth on the outside, on the inside it was irregular and "had a tail" on it. Right then, when he said that, I knew in my heart that I had breast cancer. He recommended a biopsy as soon as possible, and indicated that I needed surgery to remove it—regardless if it was cancerous or not—as soon as possible. "Within the next two weeks," was his suggestion. Then everything after that was a blur.

There was a meeting with a breast surgeon, a

very painful core needle biopsy, and the agonizing wait. We went for my follow-up with the surgeon and he told me, "We have your pathology results back, and unfortunately"—hearing THAT word, I mentally broke down—"unfortunately, it IS cancer." Then he began telling me that I could have a lumpectomy, or a mastectomy; THEN he told me that he sees a lot of younger women with breast cancer have a DOUBLE mastectomy. He then told me that the standard protocol for women my age diagnosed with breast cancer is chemotherapy. I heard that word and started bawling again. I knew what chemo meant. It meant I would lose my hair! It meant I would get sick.

"Oh God," I thought, "I AM sick. I have cancer. I have CANCER. Cancer KILLS people. What will my girls do without their mommy?"

For this appointment we left our eldest daughter with my mom. I didn't want her there if it was going to be bad news. And I was fairly certain it was going to be just that. We went home for a while to let the news sink in. I called my two best friends and told them. I had a very hard time calling my mom and telling her.

"How in the *world* can I tell my mom that I have cancer?" I asked my husband Tim. "It will devastate her."

And it did just that, to both of my parents. I made sure, though, that when I told people that I did have cancer, I told them it was the most common form, and that it was highly treatable. I didn't want everyone sad and worried about me. But, we did let everyone close to us know and, after researching my surgical options, we met with a plastic surgeon and the oncologist who would be treating me. I decided to have bi-lateral mastectomies. I would have the breast with the cancer in it completely removed, along with a few lymph nodes to check if the cancer had spread. And I would have my cancer-free breast removed as well. This would give me both peace of mind when thinking of the chance of having a second bout in the other breast *and* a better physical result with reconstruction than if I had just one breast reconstructed and had to try to match the other one with a breast reduction and lift.

I made peace with my body in the days before my surgery. I stared at them in the mirror, I took pictures in my bathing suit on my cell phone, knowing it would be the last time they'd be seen like that. I didn't want to freak out after my surgery when looking down at my chest—before, I would see my d-cup breasts that had fed both of my children, that had (in all honesty) played a part in my landing my husband. I just plain *loved* my boobs. They looked good still after two kids, and I was proud of them. But, at the same time, one of them could kill me. I wanted them BOTH out.

I handled the surgery very well. I was not in as much pain as I had anticipated and, after a nice two-night hospital vacation, I went home. My chest was bandaged up pretty tight, but I snuck glances when I could. Taking the bandages off was not the trauma I had envisioned. The scars weren't the monstrosities I thought they would be. I had "made peace" with my body in the days before my surgery. After my surgeon removed both breasts along with the lymph nodes, my plastic surgeon inserted silicone expanders under my pectoral muscles in my chest, and filled them with 120 cc's of saline. Every two weeks I would get another 100 cc's of saline injected in them until we reached my desired size. Since the implants were under my muscles, we had to use the expanders to allow for my skin and muscles to stretch to accommodate my new implants. I healed up very well, was feeling better within days, and was ready to start phase two of my cancer journey: chemotherapy. When I got the diagnosis from my doctor and he told me I would most likely need chemo, I cried even harder than when he told me I had cancer. It had just taken my breasts from me. Now it wanted my hair, too. And my eyelashes. And my eyebrows.

I have ALWAYS had self-esteem issues, and never felt like I was "pretty." And I always have felt that I was judged by my looks by everyone. I felt inferior because I had bad skin, with some scarring, and I had been teased about it a few times when I was younger. Those kids who teased me were just being kids; I understand that now as an adult, but I took it to heart way back then and it's been there ever since.

A week before I started chemo, I had an outpatient surgical procedure to have a "port" inserted under the skin in my chest, where the chemo would be administered. This was to save my veins from collapsing, and would be the easiest way to get the life-saving drugs into my body.

Then I had the Big Day: my first chemo. For most people, chemo is a community experience. You're in a room with other people, not in a hospital bed by yourself. Everyone has a comfy recliner with a little table next to it, and a fancy pole that your chemo bag hangs off of. I was always the youngest person in the chemo room by at least 20 years. I didn't mind it—most of them liked my bright pink hair (the first two treatments, at least, *before* I lost it) and my spunky attitude. And they thought I was cute. My first chemo was, in all reality, pretty easy. I felt ok during it and, aside from being more sensitive to smells, I didn't get a nauseous or sick feeling. Three days later I had the "chemo crash"; I got really tired, constipated, and emotional. And about 16 days after my first treatment, my hair started falling out.

I had been tugging at my hair ever since my first chemo, checking for the inevitable. At first, when I tugged on it, a few strands would come loose. A few days later, just touching my head would cause clumps to slip out. That was one of the hardest and scariest times of my life, watching my hair fall out. That is when the reality of your cancer sets it. Now I LOOKED sick. I had my husband shave my head when it got really thinned out. I couldn't take the helpless feeling of it falling out anymore. With each treatment, I got sicker and more exhausted, and more emotional. My eyebrows fell out. My eyelashes were gone. Even my nose hairs fell out,  so that I was constantly walking around with a runny nose. I was gaining weight from a combination of inactivity and the steroids they pumped me full of each time I had chemo. My eyes had dark circles all around them.

And then, in a strange twist of fate that I *still* have not been able to figure out, my mom was ALSO diagnosed with breast cancer. Other than a cousin, we had no family history of breast cancer. My mom's tumor was very tiny and her doctors were confident that she could be treated by just having the lump removed, followed by radiation and no chemotherapy. The cancer was removed by surgery, and the doctor also removed a couple of her lymph nodes for biopsy. Unfortunately, the first lymph node removed had cancerous cells in it, so they removed an additional 12 nodes. None of the others had cancer in them, but because the one node did, mom would now have to have chemotherapy in addition to her radiation. My

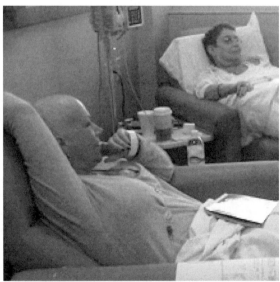

Heather and her mom, Sharon, receiving chemotherapy together

mom was so scared through everything. One thing I did notice, though, was that in immersing myself in my mom's treatment and fight against cancer, I put my own fight in the background. I was more worried about my mom than myself. And for that reason, I will forever be thankful that I was diagnosed first.

I was halfway through my treatments, I knew that it was achievable, and that cancer was not necessarily a death sentence. I could give my mom hope and take away some of her fear, and that is exactly what I did.

We even had her first few and my last few chemo treatments together, side by side. I don't know that I have ever felt as much relief as I did on the day of my last chemo treatment.

Chemotherapy has a cumulative effect, so with each treatment you get to feeling worse and worse. I gained about 17 pounds throughout chemo. I lost half of my toenails. My fingernails were getting brown spots on them and breaking off halfway down. I couldn't taste anything. My skin looked almost gray in color, my eyes had brown dark circles under them, and my eyelids were also brownish in color and puffy. My face was bloated from the steroids. I had never felt so bad before in my life, physically, but mentally I was at my peak. I was *alive!* Who gave a crap what I looked like! And for that peace of mind, for that thought—that when it comes down to it, what I look like *physically* does not change *who I am inside*—I am grateful.

It really set me free.

I finished my chemo in October, and my mom finished hers right before Christmas. She had a few weeks' break and then started her radiation therapy: five days a week for five-and-a-half weeks. Every morning she and my dad got up early to head to the cancer center across town to get her radiation therapy. She was beyond exhaustion. I went to my parents' house just about every day to spend time with my mom. I printed out information for her, brought her books and pamphlets regarding every aspect of her type of breast cancer and its treatments. Our roles had switched. I comforted *her* now. I became the caregiver.

I had read articles and heard about Hello Gorgeous! before my diagnosis and, after hearing about the organization, my mother-in-law submitted my mother and me for nomination. I was so moved by this. She even made a copy of her nomination form and gave it to me. What I did not know was that my husband had also nominated both of us to receive Hello Gorgeous! makeovers! I had NO IDEA that we had been chosen, and that Tim, my husband, had been working with Kim Becker to get my mom and me to the makeover location, all the while keeping me completely in the dark!

They ended up getting my mom and me both to a women's show at a local convention center by letting us think that a friend of my cousin was giving a speech there on cancer survival and she wanted to recognize us during her speech. They ended up having to tell my mom that I was receiving a makeover—she was feeling so bad and so tired that they had a really hard time getting mom to come. But once my dad told her I was getting a makeover, well, she would not have missed that for the world.

But she had NO idea that SHE would be getting a makeover there as well!

I was completely surprised when everyone surrounded us, gave mom and me beautiful bouquets of flowers, snapped pictures left and right, and yelled "HELLO GORGEOUS!" to us. They had their mobile DaySpa at the event, and they whisked us into that spa to begin our pampering. Mom got a manicure while I got a facial and a pedicure. Then we switched places, and I got my nails painted and mom got her facial and pedi-

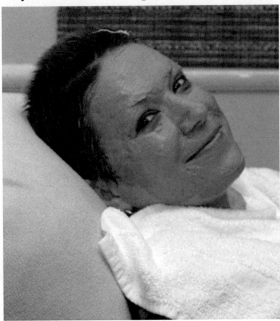

Heather in heaven during her facial

cure. We were absolutely giddy! I enjoyed seeing my mom beaming, with her big beautiful smile from ear to ear while she was being pampered. I enjoyed that just as much as I enjoyed my own pampering! The ladies who worked on us, and with us, were all so friendly and accommodating. I got my hair trimmed and some highlights put in. Since mom had just finished treatment, her hair was just beginning to come back in, so they had brought a wig for her that they trimmed and styled. The part that I'm REALLY impressed about is that Kim—the founder of Hello Gorgeous!—had been in contact with my husband and he was able to get my clothes sizes and shoe size, and my mom's as well! Without either of us knowing! Two associates from the Maurice's store in town brought bags full of clothes, shoes, and accessories for mom and me to try on. We got professional makeup applications, and were also given tips for doing it ourselves, to compensate for the damage done to our looks by the side-effects of the chemo. I had never had a makeover before but have ALWAYS wanted one. My mom and I were pampered and glammed up. We were smiling and laughing like little girls the entire time. What I didn't know was that the entire time we were in the mobile DaySpa, our family and friends were gathering for our big unveiling.

Walking onto that stage, glamorous and feeling pretty for the first time in a long time, in front of so many of our family and friends and a hundred clapping strangers at the women's show was one of the most exciting events of my life. Seeing all of my friends in the crowd, all of whom were cheering us on and applauding for us, made me feel so special and loved. It was an evening like I've never had before. The best part of it all was sharing it with my mom. We had been through so much together in the months before this, so many crappy things we had to endure, and it was such an awesome thing to do something so fun together.

We looked, and most importantly, FELT, gorgeous! We were given skincare products,

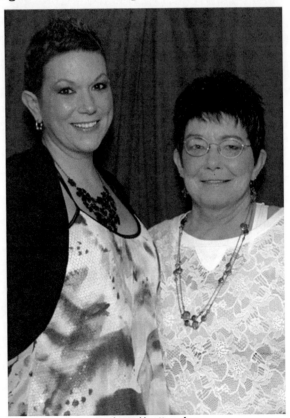

Heather and her Mom after

makeup, and clothes to take home, so we could look this way every day we needed to. It was just like Christmas! What Hello Gorgeous! did for my mom and me, making us feel so special, and giving us that experience to share with each other, went so far beyond the clothes and makeup. Thank you, girls. Thank you, Kim. We love you!

It was our first double visit in the mobile DaySpa and it was a glorious day! I will never forget their smiles and looks of wonder and I will also never forget the love I saw in the eyes of a daughter battling cancer for her mother battling cancer. What a love!

# Heather's Update

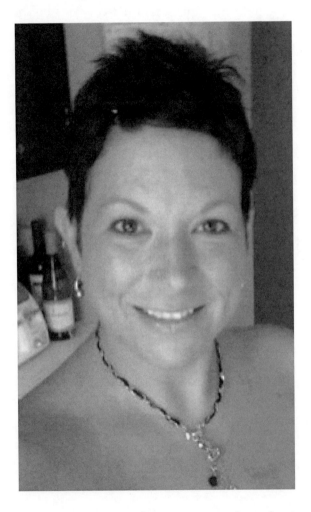

It's been a year since our diagnosis, mom's and mine. We are both in remission and plan on staying that way for a long time! It's been a long and hard journey, but I'm finally starting to feel like I'm getting back to normal. I have one more surgery coming up in September. I had genetic testing done a few months ago and found out that I am a carrier for the BRCA1 gene mutation, and being the mother of two phenomenal little girls, this scares me very much. This gene mutation is an indicator for ovarian as well as breast cancer, so my oncologist has recommended a total hysterectomy to protect me from the possibility of getting ovarian cancer in the future. I feel like I've done all that I can to fight this cancer and protect myself from a re-occurrence. I am hopeful that, by the time my daughters grow up, we will have a cure and they will never have to worry about breast cancer.

# Linda

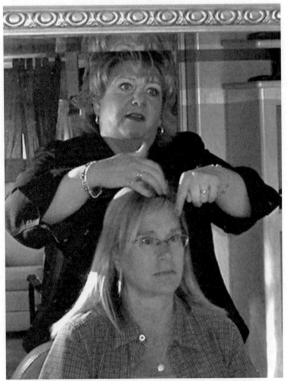

"You must be as wonderful
as my sister!"

Hello Gorgeous!

LINDA IS 49 YEARS OLD and was nominated by her sister, Patty, who sent us a wonderful letter about her sister. Patty writes:

> *"My sister should be nominated because she's in desperate need of someone to pamper her and give her a big makeover. Nine years ago, at the age of 40, shortly after giving birth to her twins, she had to have her spleen removed and was diagnosed with a slow-growing form of non-Hodgkin's lymphoma. Unfortunately, since this type usually affects elderly people, very little research has been done on it. After a series of chemo treatments, she has courageously continued to raise not only her twins, who are now nine, but also her 17- and 15-year-old children. I stay over at her home once a week to help her and her husband with the children's schoolwork, cooking dinner and catching up on laundry. But I just do not feel that I can ever do enough to help her catch up. With four children to raise, with whom she participates in all extracurricular activities as much as possible, she takes no time for herself. Her children's activities require numerous fees, which one could pay upfront or work off at various sponsors' events. She chooses the latter since her income has declined since her cancer diagnosis.*

*I was at the hospital when her doctor told her about the cancer being incurable and that it would shorten her lifespan. Even during chemo she never complained or spoke about her illness unless asked directly about it. If you met her you would not even know that she was ill or going through treatment. It's especially hard to try to explain to her children because she keeps pushing herself so hard and they don't even realize that she is ill. Although I remind her constantly that she needs to take time for herself, I think she feels that she has to pack as much into her days as possible to make up for the fact that the disease may take her away from her kids before she has done everything that she wants to do with and for them. My sister has always been the rock of the family and the one that everyone called when they needed help with anything. When my brother divorced and had his two daughters to raise, she took the time to take his daughters shopping for school clothes and guide them in the absence of their mother. When my father's Alzheimer's became advanced and he had to be placed in a nursing home, where he stayed for four-and-a-half years, she had him placed nearby her home so that she could help my mother out as much as possible. She's basically been on call for my family 24/7 for much of her life. We all came to depend on her for various things we needed help with—whether it was with taxes, babysitting, parent(s)-sitting, etc. This has all been in addition to caring for her own immediate family.*

*It is not just family that she involves herself with*

*either. She participates in all fundraisers either individually or with her kids and, most recently, was involved with the Race for the Cure, The Light of Night Lymphoma Walk, Relay for Life, and the 5K-Run for Logan Center. All the work she does is great but at the same time she does not take care of herself the way that she should and continues to work tirelessly whenever she can lend a helping hand to anyone. Hopefully her children will learn some of her generous and giving ways as they grow older. She has never let her cancer get her down until recently. In January of this year her blood tests did not look good and she will soon have to go through another round of chemo. Although her illness has never gotten her down, she has been experiencing some depression. I try to do as much as I can to help and talk to her on a daily basis, but I never feel that I can do enough. The timing of your article in the newspaper on Tuesday got me really excited. I do not feel that the time could be better for a makeover for someone who is so deserving of a little pampering and a little positive attention. She's truly a beautiful person on the inside and I would love to see that reflected on the outside as well. You can make that happen and I truly pray that you will select my sister for a makeover. God bless you for doing this for these wonderful people afflicted with this horrible disease. For all that she has done for everyone she touches in her life, she deserves to be touched by an Angel such as you and your group. Thank you for taking the*

> *time to read my letter. You must be as wonderful*
> *as my sister."*

So we chose Linda's nomination which also was done on our six-week tour, although we did this in South Bend before we left. Patty took her sister Linda to Applebee's on Ireland Road. We set the mobile DaySpa up in the restaurant parking lot an hour before Linda was scheduled to arrive and watched from the DaySpa as she walked in. We waited until the scheduled time and then went in after her. They were sitting at a table, about to order, when we stormed in with candy and flowers and a big "Hello Gorgeous!" and let Linda know that she had been nominated for a day of beauty and that she had been chosen. Linda admitted that she was disappointed to see on the 11:00 p.m. news the previous night that we had chosen a winner for the makeover and that it was not her! Wrong! We whisked her out to the mobile DaySpa sitting and she wore a Hollywood smile and had a swagger in her step as she walked the red carpet to the door and stepped inside.

Linda told us that she had been diagnosed with Non-Hodgkin's Lymphoma shortly after her twins were born. Then, within a few short months, Linda went on maternity leave, her position was eliminated from Honeywell, she was diagnosed with her cancer and her husband lost his job. On top of all this, Linda was told that *they would have to wait for her cancer to get worse before she could be treated*! Because of the four children and losing her job shortly after she had her twins, doing any extras for herself was not anything she had been used to doing. We were able to give her an entire afternoon of pampering. We gave her a pedicure, manicure and a facial. We did her makeup. We waxed her eyebrows. And we were able to cut and highlight Linda's hair.

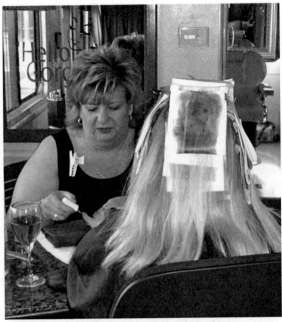

Kim giving Linda her manicure in the DaySpa

Dress Barn helped us fit her with a new outfit. Trisha from the South Bend store generously donated a $100 gift card to Linda, quizzed her on her clothing likes and dislikes, and then Trisha and Linda's sister Patty went shopping for a stunning new outfit.

She looked like she felt—phenomenal! But we were not through yet. We told Linda that she had some people waiting for her so Mike escorted her back down the red carpet and she waited in the alcove as I introduced myself to her gathered friends and the rest of the restaurant patrons. We asked everyone in Applebee's to give Linda a big "HELLO GORGEOUS!" and, as she walked in, she was very surprised to see 25 of her family members and closest friends waiting to celebrate her new look with her! It was wonderful to see her beam and they welcomed her with warm embraces. What a great night!

She just looked completely different, completely relaxed and you could see the sparkle back in her eyes. Since her visit in June of last year we've run into her several times in town and she's kept up her look and her hair is styled the same way. We certainly had a positive effect on her that day and we know that she's going to be able to beat this thing. Great job, Linda!

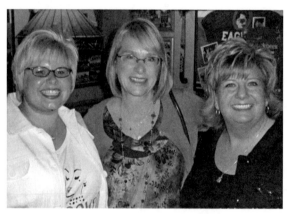

Trisha, Linda and Kim at Linda's Reveal

## Linda's Update————————————

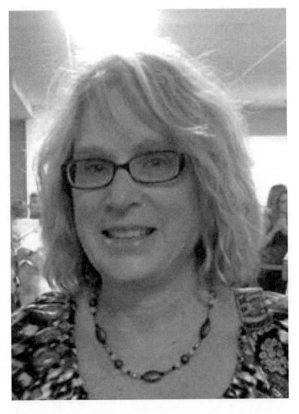

Victim. That was what I was until my experience with the wonderful people of Hello Gorgeous! "Survivor" is a popular and celebrated word in the cancer glossary but I didn't feel like a survivor and I definitely didn't look or sound like one. Sure I was alive but I felt threatened. I was a victim not a survivor—yet. I needed a moment, a life-changing event to reach survivorship and that hadn't happened with the last chemotherapy treatment or the latest blood test or CAT scan results.

Hello Gorgeous! gave me that experience. Kim, Trisha and Mike not only helped me change my outside appearance but they gave me the courage to celebrate, to be a survivor. Their kindness and charity created the transition point I so desperately needed and I will be forever grateful that our worlds collided.

# Christina

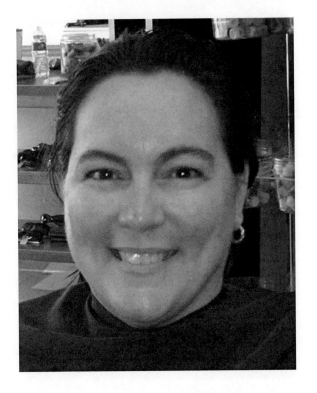

## Phenomenal Woman

Hello Gorgeous!

CHRISTINA WORKS AT A LOCAL BANK with my sister and was diagnosed in December of 2008 with breast cancer.

This is the e-mail I received from Christina:

*"Hi Kim, I'm Christina and I work with your sister Amy at the bank; she gave me your brochures and said to contact you and that both of you had talked about me recently. I started my first chemo yesterday and I receive so much information that it's all a bit overwhelming. I'm losing my hair soon and I want to keep on top of it if I can. I need to cut my hair but I'm afraid to; but I'm even more afraid of it falling out before I'm ready. I know it's going to happen but it's still not the same. I don't even know where to begin with wigs. I don't usually wear makeup but have been told maybe I should a little. I know that you don't know me but maybe we can get together soon so that I can see what your business can do to help me. I have a very busy schedule, as probably do you, so here is mine. My husband and I have a three-year-old who is a big handful right now and he's too young to understand why I don't feel good. Let me know if you can help me. Thanks, Christina."*

We got that e-mail on a Friday. My sister Trish and I decided that Christina needed our help so we contacted her and asked her if she could meet us at the salon on Sunday. That next Sunday we decided it wasn't enough for us just to help her with her hair. We were going to do a full-out visit on her that day, only she didn't know it. Here is Christina's story, in her own words:

"Just when you think you have improved your life and you are very happy, things can change in an instant. This story will start from the point where I was very happy and how we have struggled the past few years. By we, I have to include my husband as he also has felt some of the pain and then some of his own too. After getting together with my high school sweetheart after a divorce, I never thought I would marry again. I married Bill in August of 2002, which was the highlight of my life. It was the happiest time of my life when our son Louis was born in June of 2005. We had discussed having two children besides the step-children we both already had; however, the Lord must have had other plans for us.

In June of 2007, we received news that I was pregnant. Things seemed to be going fine, but when we went to my doctor appointment in August, the doctors could not find a heartbeat. They ordered an ultrasound and determined that I had lost the baby. Bill and I were both devastated. I had never been through anything like this but, with both of us embracing each other like never before, we were able to get through it. We continued to try, and a few months later I went to a routine doctor appointment in December and was told I was pregnant again, the week before Christmas. Have you ever had so much excitement—thinking that the Lord wanted to surprise you to give you another blessing? But in receiving this unexpected news, I was to be devastated the same day learning that I had miscarried again. I kept thinking we would not be able to have another child, as I was getting closer to 40 years old.

In 2008 Bill had some medical issues and needed to have surgery. I had just had a mammogram, suggested by my family doctor, since I had just turned 40. And it was while at the University of Chicago Hospital, as I walked out of Bill's pre-op when the nurses were taking him to begin a five-hour surgery, that my cell phone rang. It was my family doctor's nurse telling me they found a mass in the ultrasound of my mammogram on the right breast. She said I needed to have a diagnostic mammogram done soon. I sat in the surgical waiting room for five hours, scared and worried, knowing there was no one to talk to. I was alone in Chicago. I called my mom and she calmed me down, telling me she has had fatty tissue masses for years and my mass was probably something like that. I was still scared and wanting the second ultrasound done right now! When I was in Bill's room, waiting for recovery to bring him in, I talked to his nurse. She said she would say prayers for both of us. I wish I could remember her name because I have never had a stranger show so much understanding as she. She not only took care of my husband, she also cared about what I was going through. I thank her for that and I will never forget it.

A week later I went in for the diagnostic mammogram. My nurse Rita was another blessing. She made sure I was very comfortable and explained everything that was going to happen. The doctor read the pictures right on the spot and suggested that I needed a biopsy. He thought the mass did not look cancerous, but it did look "different" and they wanted to be sure.

The week before Thanksgiving I went in for the biopsy and was told they would have results in a week or two because of the holiday. By the end of the first week in December I hadn't heard anything so Rita made another call for me. Come to find out that our own lab could not make the diagnosis and they had sent it to another University to make the diagnosis. It was a rainy, cold and just downright ugly day in the second week in December. Just after I came into work I received a phone call from my family doctor. He told me that, with the inclement weather, he would talk to me on the phone with the news. He told me over the phone, right at my desk at work, the results of the biopsy and that I had breast cancer. I will never forget that day—at work for Pete's sake! I confided in my supervisor and said I'd be back in a while. I needed to collect myself. I went out into the foyer and called my husband, of course, crying and very upset.

I was angry that I was told at work. I was in disbelief that I had breast cancer. How could this have happened to me? There is no history of it in my family at all. "Why me?" kept going through my mind. When I told my mother and my entire family they were as shocked as I was.

My family doctor then referred me to Dr. Thomas, who scheduled me for surgery on December 19. The surgery went great. Dr. Thomas had removed all of the mass, cleaned the margins and also removed five lymph nodes. In January, I was scheduled to see an oncologist who would tell me everything that I would need to do and the results of the mass. I had so many questions and concerns. The first thing she wanted to do was put me in a clinical trial and they would send samples of my mass to the University of California to study whether or not I would have a high chance of re-occurrence for the cancer. They tested whether my cancer was ER and/or PR positive, determining whether or not I would have to have chemotherapy. I was sure that I wouldn't have to, but two weeks later I was called and told my score was very high and I would have to have chemotherapy and radiation. And then came the most devastating news . . . We would not be able to have any more children.

My doctor wanted to start chemo the following week. I asked for the chemo to begin later in the week as I needed to make sure things at work would be okay and that I would miss the least amount of time possible. All I could think about was that we could have no more children, and that was I going to lose my hair. I cried myself to sleep most nights for a week or so. Bill tried to comfort me but he was scared for me too. He held me tight every night.

News spread fast around work that I was go-ing to have chemo. One of the ladies in another department told me to talk with a gal named Amy who worked in the same building, because her sister had started an organization that might be able to help me. I didn't know anything about this organization called Hello Gorgeous!

Thursday was "Chemo Day," sounding too much like "D-Day" to me. Bill and I went to the infusion lab and a new friend, Kim Z, showed up as well, just after they hooked up the IV. Bill sat down right next to me, but I was hungry and so Bill decided to walk to McDonald's to get us something to eat. Kim sat down to be there with me and then Nurse Andrea came over and started the first drug, Taxotier.

She told me if I feel anything different at all, like numbness in my hands, to let her know right away. Kim and I continued to talk and I felt a little pain in my stomach, but I thought I was just hungry. Within seconds, the pain moved and got worse. Kim went to get the nurse and, by the time they looked over at me, I could not breathe and I was turning red. They ran back to me and Nurse Andrea called out different things to the other nurses there STAT. I was totally scared and wanted them to stop everything but I couldn't talk. Of course Bill showed up *after* all the excitement! I had a very bad reaction to the drug, a one-in-a-million chance. After about five hours, long enough for them to pump the drugs in very slowly because of the reaction, we finally went home.

I didn't work on Friday, not knowing how I was going to feel, so I took that time to call Kim. She asked me to email pictures of myself to her and explain how I wear my hair. She asked me to meet her at her salon late Sunday morning.

I awoke Sunday not feeling very well at all. I made it to the salon with my husband's help and my son Louis came along. We all walked in together not knowing what to expect and, to our surprise, we were greeted by Kim and Trish with roses and candy and a big "Hello Gorgeous!" I told them I wasn't feeling very well and Kim told me everything they had planned for me. If I wasn't comfortable or needed to stop I was to let them know. I didn't know what to expect. I did not even know what it was going to cost me!

Trish started out giving me a facial; I had never had one done before and it made me feel very relaxed. Afterward Kim gave me a massage. I had told her that my back was very sore so she started out very slowly and gently. It was also my first massage and it was wonderful. I didn't want it to end because it felt so good and my pain was going away as well. But all good things must come to an end.

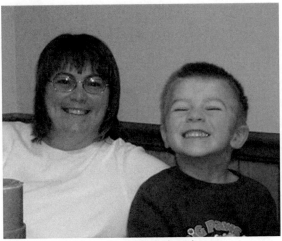

Christina and her son, Louis, during her visit

It was now time for a pedicure and manicure. During these they told me important things, like not to use a razor on my legs right now because I didn't want any kind of infection if I were to nick myself. They were using nail files and no clippers, so I would not get any open wounds. Next it was time to transition me to a shorter haircut, for when I started losing my hair. Kim gave me the cutest cut and after the cut we tried on some wigs. I could not believe how much fun my family had seeing those different hairstyles on me! Trish went to get a hat that I could wear when I lost my hair. It was so soft! I chose a pink one, of course, but my son Louis loved it so much he tried on a black one himself. We all laughed, as he looked so cute, and we had to get the camera for a picture. We picked out a wig (and Kim held on to it for me until I lost my hair). Trish then showed me how to put on makeup again, to help hide the fact I would have no eyelashes or eyebrows during chemotherapy. I had never been shown how to put makeup on before. She gave me a bag with all the makeup items in it that she used on me and told me it was mine to keep and use. Wow!! What a wonderful day! I had never been pampered like these two ladies pampered me in my entire life.

We all had a blast. After it was over, I asked how much I owed them and I was told "nothing." They just wanted to make me feel better. It was the most gracious thing anyone has ever done for me. We hugged and cried.

I received a call a week later from Kim Z asking me how I was doing.

"Well, I have not lost any hair yet," I said. "Yeah!!" But the following week, as I sat in a meeting at work, I ran my fingers through my hair and a handful came out. The next day it was worse. I called Kim Z and told her I didn't know how much more I could take. It was time to cut it off. She told me she would call me right back and to stay by my phone. When she called she said that she, Kim, and I would need to be at the salon on Sunday. That Sunday was Super Bowl Sunday. At least it wasn't Valentine's Day.

We arrived at 10 a.m. and started talking. I sat in the chair and Kim Becker gently took off my glasses. She pulled out an electric razor, just like the one I use on my husband's hair, and started shaving my head. She used the number 4 guard on the razor (I'll never forget it) and turned me away from the mirror, so that I did not have to watch. She was soon done and I asked Kim Z for my glasses and asked Kim Becker to turn me around. I wanted to see myself. I was shocked, not at having no hair, but that I looked just like my dad! They all laughed with me for a while as Kim tried on the wig we picked out. She trimmed it up around my face and combed it out, explained to me how to wash and care for it, and gave me products to take care of it as well. We took pictures when we were finished, said our goodbyes to our new friends, and headed home.

I stood alone in front of the mirror for a while in disbelief when we got home. This had really happened to me. Wow. I knew that if I got through this I could get through anything. My personality is one of joy. I am always full of smiles unless I'm in pain or upset. I would say 95% of the time I'm smiling. I told myself I needed to keep that attitude to get through the next six months. So much had been taken away from me, the worst being my dreams of having more children. I thank God every day for letting me get through those tough few years. I now devote as much of my spare time to helping Hello Gorgeous! as I can. I tell people about them and enjoy attending the different functions they have.

In August of 2010 my hair had grown back enough that I called Kim to see if she could cut my hair. She trimmed it and we talked about color when it got a little longer. A few months later I chose a red color, and with my short hair and red color I looked like my brothers, who are both redheads.

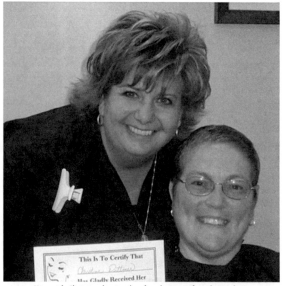

Kim with Christina having her first haircut after chemotherapy

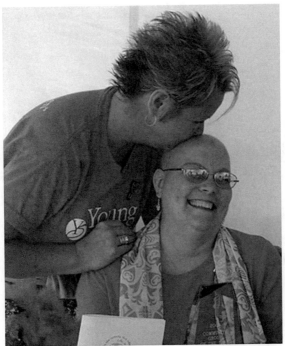

Christina getting a kiss on the head from her friend Kim Z

In November 2009 I was chosen as the 2010 Gorgeous! Ambassador for Hello Gorgeous! I enjoyed helping them at many of their events and we also participated in the parades they and the mobile DaySpa were in. The most fun was their big event in November, the Comedy Luncheon. And to this day I still enjoy helping them and telling my story.

Thank you, Kim, Mike, and Trish. I will be forever in your debt. I believe that each one of you has a heart of gold and, now that you have Affiliate Salons to help you, a lot more women will be helped like I was.

Your upbeat, positive and happy Gorgeous Gal, Christina

Throughout Christina's treatment, she did a wonderful job with wearing different hats and scarves and the wig that we had gotten her. There were days that I would catch her out and about when she would just have a bald head with her hat on top of it. She's an amazing inspiration.

Christina has become a great friend. She was our 2010 Gorgeous! Ambassador for Hello Gorgeous! and she has done wonderful things for our community. The smile and the spark that this horrible diagnosis has put into her has been a wonderful transformation to see. Nothing in life gets

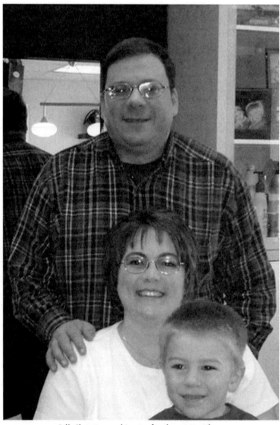

Bill, Christina and Louis after her visit with us

her down now and she just doesn't take things for granted. She's completely back where she was; if you didn't know that she had breast cancer you would not be able to tell. What an amazing inspiration and what a wonderful way to allow something negative to empower you. Christina is an amazing woman.

# Christina's Update———————————

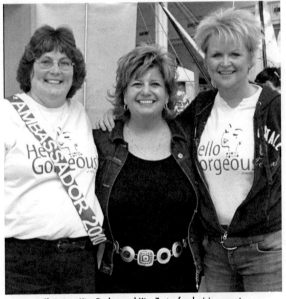

Christina, Kim Becker and Kim Z at a fundraising event

## What It Has Meant to Be the Ambassador for Hello Gorgeous!

When I was nominated to be the Gorgeous! Ambassador of Hello Gorgeous! I wasn't sure what it meant. I only knew I wanted to help them in any way I could. Being a cancer survivor, I just want to tell everyone that early detection is the answer because not everyone's lump is detected by self-examination. Mine was only detected by mammogram.

My first mammogram was in October of 2008 at age 40; by the end of January, I was facing chemo and was scared to death. With the help of Hello Gorgeous! I had the courage to face anything that came my way. My positive attitude also helped. When I was nominated Ambassador, the first event I was a part of was a surprise and reveal for another woman on St. Patrick's Day. The atmosphere was electrifying with so many people attending an enjoyable evening. I enjoyed walking in the parades. Some people had heard of Hello Gorgeous! and some had not, so in passing out the brochures I know I'm doing my part in getting the word out about the organization. Being a finalist in Mutual of Omaha's "Aha Moment" contest was also exciting even though I didn't make it to the final round.

Thank you, Kim, for all you do to make cancer patients feel whole again, for making a life-altering experience a way for me to look back and say it wasn't so bad and I had very good friends to help me get through it.

*Christina Dettman,*
Hello Gorgeous! Ambassador 2010

# Kathy

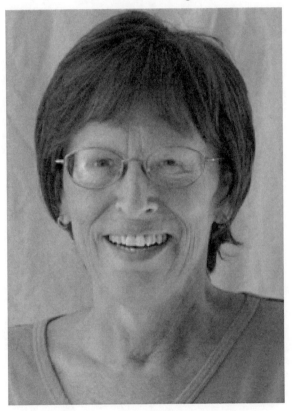

"It's all good!"

# Hello Gorgeous!

I WANT TO TELL YOU ONE OF MY FAVORITE STORIES, about a beautiful Gorgeous Woman by the name of Kathy. Kathy was a visit we did in Muncie, Indiana, on our tour in July of 2010.

As we were going throughout the state of Indiana we wanted to introduce the Hello Gorgeous! Experience to the different parts of the state. I didn't necessarily know people to get in touch with to find a candidate in Muncie, so Katie, the assistant marketing director at Muncie Mall, actually had a friend who had recently been diagnosed with breast cancer. This friend was Kathy.

Here is her nomination:

> *"Kathy is such a hard-working, loving, energetic and humorous woman. She's a mother, wife, grandmother and daughter. I worked with Kathy and got to witness sadly her being diagnosed with breast cancer just months before her daughter graduated from high school. Without insurance, this has been a long, hard battle for Kathy and her family. Kathy does not miss a day of work except for chemo and continues to stay as positive as she can. She continually says life is good, with a smile on her face. Also Kathy does not spend any money on herself, to pamper herself in any way. She currently has one wig to cover her bald head. I believe she deserves this gracious act in order to give her and her family hope."*

Katie helped us arrange getting Kathy to the mall so that we could surprise her. Kathy was inside Bath and Body Works at the Muncie Mall thinking that she was just shopping for the day. We showed up unannounced inside Bath and Body Works, presented her with candy and flowers, and we had a big banner that said *"Hello Gorgeous!"*

We let her know that she had been nominated for a day of beauty and that she had been chosen. The look on her face was priceless. She had no clue what was happening. She kept saying to us, "Now what's really going on? What's *really* going on here?" We explained it to her again that she'd been nominated for this day of beauty and that she'd been chosen. We escorted her outside the mall where we had the red carpet rolled out, escorted her onto the mobile DaySpa, and told her a little bit about what her day would include.

It was one of our best makeovers ever.

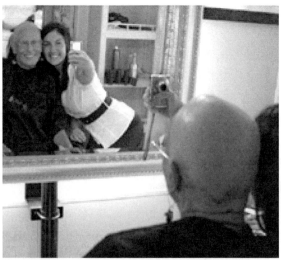

Kathy and Katie, Assistant Marketing Director of Muncie Mall

We were fortunate enough to contact Kathy about writing about her own experience for us for this book and she was excited to do so. Weeks later, Mike and I heard that

Kathy had a recurrence of cancer in her brain and was in the hospital, not doing well. And in an instant, it seemed, we received a call to say that Kathy was gone. Here are Kathy's own words about her experience with us:

"It started out as a normal Saturday in July 2010 and turned into a fabulous day! A small group of friends and my daughter Chelsi had planned a shopping trip to the Muncie Mall. We were in the Bath and Body Works store and I was busy trying out free samples when all of a sudden a large group from Hello Gorgeous! including Kim, Trisha and their wonderful team came right up to me. They were saying "Hello Gorgeous!" to me and I looked around to make sure they were talking to me. I was feeling not-too-gorgeous at that time because cancer treatment takes a toll on you.

They presented me with candy, flowers and a framed certificate. I was escorted out of the store and through the mall on the arm of a young man named Dan, then out of the mall entirely and out into the mobile DaySpa and the transformation began. It all started out with physical changes but by that afternoon my whole attitude was transformed. The entire time they kept giving me positive information and made me feel so much better. They are such a kind and loving group to be involved with. They changed my life and gave me some wonderful memories to cherish and a new group of friends.

The complete video of this event can be seen on YouTube. Just type in the search: Hello Gorgeous New York Experience 2010.

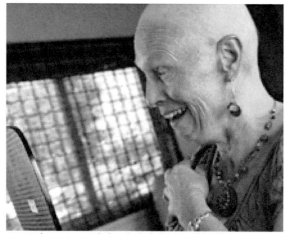
Kathy was surprised when she looked at herself for the first time

When I think of my friends from Hello Gorgeous! it makes me smile just remembering that day. I had been fighting cancer since March 2010 and so, by July, I was not feeling too gorgeous. But by that afternoon I was feeling wonderful, thanks to this group.

The makeover included a facial, new makeup, a pedicure, manicure and polish, a new wig and new clothes from head to toes. The clothes included shoes, jeans, camisole, top, purse and jewelry, compliments of the wonderful people of Maurice's Clothing. I would never have been able to purchase these extravagant things due to all the medical bills we have. I truly felt spoiled and special that day. I am so thankful for this wonderful group and am so happy they could bless other cancer patients with their caring and love.

At the Reveal at the restaurant I truly did feel GORGEOUS as I was escorted from the DaySpa, down the red carpet and into the restaurant where

I had no idea that friends, family and co-workers were waiting for me. They could not believe how fabulous I looked and neither could I.

On November 6, 2010, Hello Gorgeous! held their annual fundraiser event called the "Gorgeous Gals Comedy Luncheon" in South Bend, Indiana. I was honored to be invited to attend as an inspirational speaker. What a great day that was and I was happy to tell my makeover story

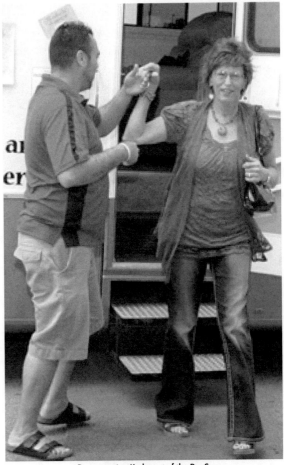

Dan escorting Kathy out of the DaySpa

in the hopes of inspiring other cancer patients, survivors and their families. They actually had the DaySpa INSIDE the convention center where another team of Makeover Specialists did a makeover on another woman during the show. It was wonderful to see the transformation and, when she stepped out in view of the crowd, the smile on her face was all too familiar to how I felt that day in July. What a memory.

I am still talking to everyone who will listen about my Hello Gorgeous! Experience and how it changed my life. This is a wonderful group of people that continues to share the love and kindness by traveling around improving the lives of cancer patients everywhere. I am truly blessed to know them."

What I remember more than anything about Kathy's visit was the transformation in her. It was not about the manicure or the pedicure; it was about watching an internal transformation take place. She went from this meek and mild, un-empowered woman faced with cancer back to someone

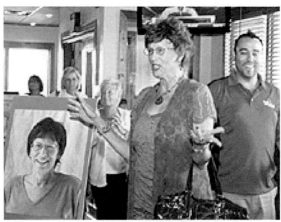

Kathy strutting her stuff at her Reveal Party

who, when we got her to her Reveal Party, was walking in and "strutting her stuff." We were able to give her back her fire, so that when the reveal crowd greeted her by yelling, "Hello Gorgeous!" she looked at everyone and said, *"I knew you were talking to me!"*

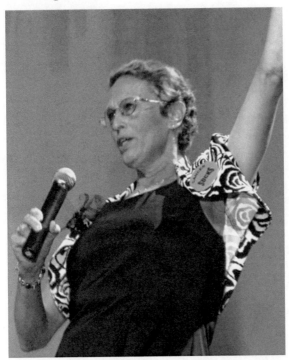

Kathy speaking at the Comedy Luncheon

We had the honor of having professional photographers with us that day. They captured everything on film and seeing the pictures of her transformation is absolutely amazing.

Kathy came to our event in November of 2010 and was our inspirational speaker. We also awarded her our yearly inspirational award because of the way that she fought her battle. Her common phrase to us was, *"It's good, it's all good."* We knew that her doctors were going to do a few more chemotherapy treatments and she had told the crowd at the November event that she knew she would lose her hair again but that was okay. It was okay because she had been through that before and her statement was, and I believed this with all my heart, *"I can kick cancer's ass."*

God's Speed, Kathy. We will never forget you.

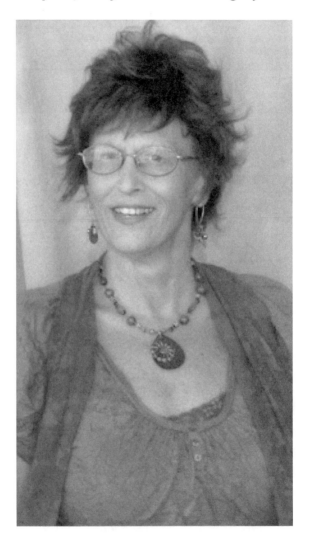

# Kay

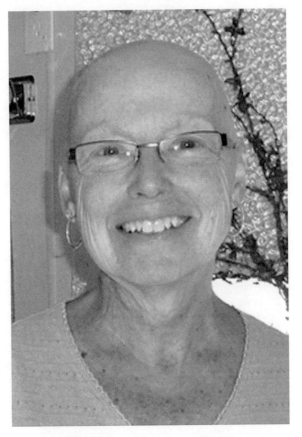

"She Is Our Glue"

### Hello Gorgeous!

AFTER WE RECEIVED THIS NOMINATION from her daughter-in-law, Missy, and Kay's children, we just had to help her.

**From Missy:** *" 'Why do you feel that this woman should be nominated and how would our services benefit her?' When I first read this question, a million different reasons ran through my mind as I tried to sort through all the numerous ways that I thought Kay would benefit from the services. I wondered how I would ever decide what to include in this nomination. Then suddenly it dawned on me that there were other people who could answer this question far more exclusively than I ever could, and those are her four children. I believe that this provides a more comprehensive understanding of how the Hello Gorgeous! services would benefit Kay and the overall value that it would bring to their entire family. Thank you for providing such a wonderful service to our local and extended community."*

**From her son Jason:** *"I will never forget the day that my mother told me that she had cancer. She told me that she always knew there was a history of cancer in our family and that meant that there was a good possibility that she might get cancer one day. Regardless, she told me that when the doctor tells you that he thinks you actually have cancer it is no longer theoretical. It is completely different and it is scary. From that moment until* *now, four chemotherapy treatments later, she has faced ups and downs, happy days and sick days, hopes and fears. But she has taken it all in stride, putting on a brave face so that the rest of the family could feel confident and put on their own brave faces. Even through these roughest of times, my mom thinks more about her family than herself. I would like to nominate my mother for a Hello Gorgeous! Experience so that she can stop thinking of others first for a short time and simply take time out for herself. She is a gorgeous person inside and out right now, but this experience would be a wonderful gift to help her rejuvenate her spirits, to be pampered and build her confidence to face the remainder of her treatments and conquer this disease."*

**Her son Aaron wrote**: *"Every family has a person that is the glue of their group. It wasn't until my mom found out about her cancer that I realized that she is our glue. My mom is a wonderfully beautiful person inside and out. She has always put her kids and family before herself. If you look at our family albums, she's rarely in them because she is always taking the pictures of the people that she loves so much. My mom has always been our biggest supporter throughout all of our endeavors and the shoulder to cry on during our toughest times. My mom is the reason that her family feels like a family. When someone has been the "rock" for so many people for so long, it's especially tough for that person to be the one in need. The Hello Gorgeous! organization can help my mom feel gorgeous again even during her time of need* *and it can help her understand that others are there to help during her time of need as well."*

**Her daughter Stephanie wrote:** *"Back in February when we found out that my mom might have cancer, I felt like my life was falling apart. It wasn't until a couple weeks later when she was officially diagnosed that I was at a complete loss for the first time in my life. I've always had mom there to help me, guide me and point me in the right direction. But here was uncharted territory for all of us and I never imagined how much one word, cancer, can change lives instantly. I knew that I now needed to step up, along with the rest of the family, to be the rock that my mom has always been for us. In the beginning mom tried to continue to be the strong one and to help the rest of us cope with the disease instead of letting us help her. It wasn't until after my mom's hair started falling out that she said, "I guess that there's no pretending that I'm not sick." My mom is the most beautiful person I know, inside and out. She has such a kind heart and a love for life that she has touched more lives than I can even count. She's not only the best mom but in her life she has played many roles that she has thrown herself into wholeheartedly including wife, daughter, sister, teacher, and friend. I think this makeover will help mom realize that even though she is going through this, she is not alone."*

**Her daughter Ashley wrote:** *"Recently my mom was diagnosed with lymphoma—cancer—a word that I never imagined crossing my mind as something that I'd have to use to describe my* *mom. She has always been the strongest person in our family. She made it to every game, every band camp, dance recital, school event, wedding, shower and more. She not only did this for all four kids but she did it for my dad and for all of her grandkids as well. She tried to never miss a thing. She did everything in the world to support us and let us know that we all were loved.*

*Now it is our turn. I want my mom to know how beautiful she is and always has been. It's my turn to be strong for her. She is the greatest woman, and knowing her strength she will make it out better and even more beautiful in the end. Each day it takes a lot of strength for her to get out of bed and pull herself together. This amazing service will allow someone else to pamper her and care for her like she did for each of us. I'm truly blessed to have such an amazing mother and best friend and I want her to feel just as loved and beautiful as she has made us feel every day of our lives."*

We performed Kay's visit on August 13, 2010. We pulled the mobile DaySpa in front of her house and rolled the red carpet out and up onto their driveway. Her daughter-in-law, daughter and two very good friends were there with us waiting for her. We showed up at the front door, knocked on the door, and when she opened it we greeted her with *"Hello Gorgeous!"* and let her know that she was nominated for a day of beauty and that she had been chosen.

We escorted her into the mobile DaySpa and had a wonderful afternoon filled with all the spa services: manicure, pedicure, facial, massage. Then we did her makeup and found her a wig. Throughout the entire day her daughter,

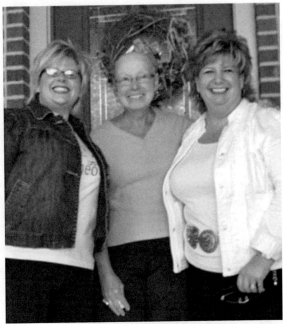

Trisha and Kim surprising Kay at her front door

daughter-in-law and her two friends stayed with us inside the mobile DaySpa. Inside the house, her husband was making cocktails and appetizers that he would deliver on a regular basis to the DaySpa on the driveway. It was quite an experience. She was just an amazing woman and you could tell how much she was loved by her family.

After her visit we received a thank you note:

"Kim, I can't begin to thank you and Trisha for all the pampering that you gave Kay a few weeks ago and for all of the help from Mike and Seth. Honestly the timing couldn't have been more perfect. After dealing with Kay's diagnosis and several family deaths the past couple of months, this was the first positive situation that we had in a long time and one that was welcomed with open arms. Kay was glowing the whole day and it was the most I've seen her smile in quite some time.

We did go to Granite City and celebrated her new look with some food and drinks. Ironically, the lady that waited on us was also working there the day you kicked off the Hello Gorgeous! tour, so she knew all about it and was very complimentary. What a great idea to have pictures being updated on Facebook throughout the day. It was a huge benefit to keeping Kay's daughter in San Diego as

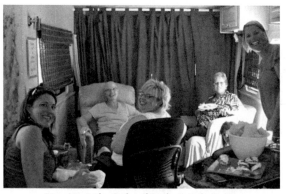

Missy, Kay, Trisha, Cindy and Stephanie in the DaySpa

well as all other close family members and friends connected with her Hello Gorgeous! Experience."

Kay updated her Caring Bridge site a couple of days later and shared her pampering day with others, so I thought that it would be rewarding for you to hear what she said in her own words:

"Friday, August 13, I was greeted with the words "Hello Gorgeous!" My children nominated me for a day of pampering that this organization provides for cancer patients and survivors. They arrived at my door with flowers, chocolate and a red carpet leading into a mobile DaySpa. My daughter Stephanie, daughter-in-law Missy, and friends Peg and Cindy were here to share in the surprise. I was treated to a facial, manicure, pedicure, makeup, a beautiful new wig and a new outfit with jewelry to match.

I was also given a gift card to one of my favorite restaurants so we all went out to lunch. Steve added to the day by providing everyone with drinks and snacks. What a day! This organization—Hello Gorgeous!—is run by a local family and they volunteer all of their time. They were wonderful and their commitment to help restore a cancer patient's mind and spirit is amazing. You undoubtedly have a gift that keeps on giving. We are blessed to have experienced what you do and see firsthand how much you give back to the community. The two words "thank you," no matter how vibrantly I say them, can't express well enough the gratitude and appreciation I have for your talent and kind-heartedness. Thank you for being such a wonderful inspiration to others."

# Kay's Update

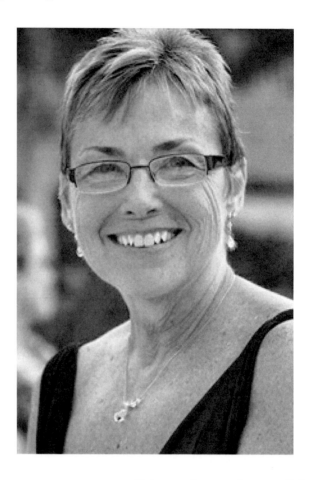

Today, my cancers are still in remission. I am still feeling healthy and even walked four miles in this year's Cancer Survivor's Walk in Chicago, Illinois, before traveling to the Dominican Republic for my daughter's wedding. Now that is what feeling good and making the most of every day is all about!

# Cindy

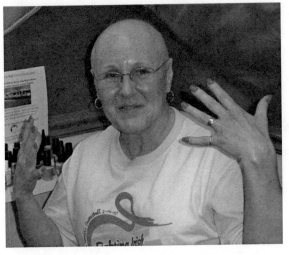

I Wish Every Day Could Be
A Hello Gorgeous! Day

Hello Gorgeous!

Cindy was nominated by her friend Marilyn and is a Red Hat lady. Cindy had been diagnosed with breast cancer and she came to our visit with two of her friends, Karen and Marilyn. I asked Marilyn to write a little bit about what it was like to watch her friend receive these services. Here's what she wrote:

"HELLO GORGEOUS! Cancer is an event in a woman's life unlike any other. Being a two-time cancer survivor, I know what it's like to go through treatment and feel less than attractive as a woman. So when I heard that Cindy had breast cancer for the second time, I wanted to step up and help her any way that I could. Cindy and I are Red Hat sisters and have spent a lot of time together in group activities. I really got to know Cindy's heart during the time we spent together in her chemotherapy treatments.

Cindy is a beautiful person who loves to help other people. She works with the United Cancer Fund of Elkhart County to raise money, mostly through a yearly cancer run/walk, so that financial aid can be given to cancer patients to help with day-to-day expenses (incurred in addition to treatment costs) as well as providing mammograms for those women who cannot afford them. To help you understand her generosity, a few years ago Cindy also organized a spaghetti luncheon at Coachmen RV, the company where she worked.

She made all the spaghetti and sauce herself and enlisted the help of family members and friends to provide other food items. The event raised hundreds of dollars for the United Cancer Fund.

Cindy and her friend also play Mrs. Clause and Santa for friends and organizations at various holiday functions, and it was during that time that someone gave her the card with the web address of Hello Gorgeous! Cindy handed it to me and asked, "Do you know what this is?" I'd previously heard of Hello Gorgeous! through news reports on the television and I let the card linger in my purse for a few weeks, and then was prodded by my consciousness to contact Kim Becker.

She provided the necessary details to nominate Cindy and I guess the rest is history. Cindy

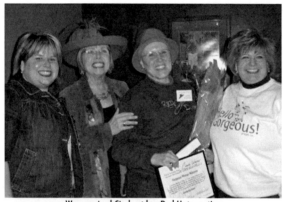
We surprised Cindy at her Red Hat meeting

has given so much to others that I wanted to do something for her. By this time she had lost her hair and was feeling a little down to say the least. She had had several chemo treatments by that time followed by a double mastectomy.

Kim, Mike and Trish surprised Cindy at a Red

Hat meeting at Michael's Restaurant in Elkhart on a snowy, cold January night. Mike walked in unannounced and said, "Hello Gorgeous!" to Cindy, while Kim and Trish presented her with a bouquet of flowers, candy and a certificate for her day of beauty. Cindy was totally overwhelmed and dissolved into tears along with the rest of us. She had no idea of the fantastic experience that was awaiting her. Cindy booked an appointment on a Friday, which turned out to be a beautiful sunny day in February and highly unusual for northern Indiana in the winter.

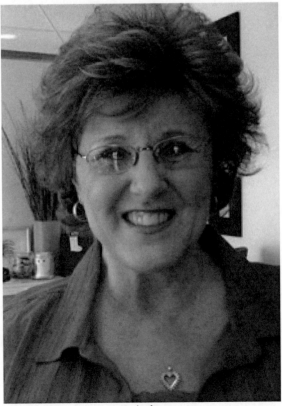

Cindy after

Kim and Trisha greeted us with big smiles that stayed on their faces throughout the day. What fun they are to be around! Cindy was treated to a wig cut and style, facial, massage, manicure, pedicure, makeover and even new sunglasses. Cindy even got to take home the hair and makeup products that were used on her during her makeover. And she was given great beauty advice from Trish throughout the day.

Cindy couldn't stop smiling! She was treated like a queen with everyone's attention focused on

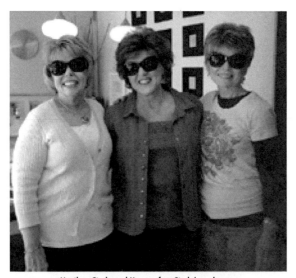

Marilyn, Cindy and Karen after Cindy's makeover

her. Cindy looked absolutely stunning. We had such a great time sharing the experience with her and we were always made to feel welcome and a part of that big day. I think that we had as much fun watching Cindy as she had receiving it. We took pictures throughout the day to document the wonderful experience and of course, since Cindy was so gorgeous, we just *had* to go out to eat. Trisha and Kim quizzed us about where we were going to eat and when we got there another surprise was waiting for us. As the three of us walked into the Granite City restaurant, the manager greeted us with "Hello Gorgeous!" and offered us an appetizer on the house!

What a perfect ending to a wonderful day! As we left the restaurant, the sun was shining brightly. Cindy and the rest of us were wearing our new sunglasses and I believe Cindy truly felt like a star.

Each time Cindy shares the story of her awesome day with a friend, she is reduced to tears at that wonderful memory. We made a photo album of pictures taken that day along with captions so that Cindy can relive that experience with her friends who were not able to be there. Her words for Kim and Trisha are just awesome. I wish every Friday could be a Hello Gorgeous! day. Cindy is keeping up with her new makeup routine and she loves wearing her newly styled wig. The experience was incredibly uplifting for Cindy and, in spite of daily issues that arise from her treatments and just making it from day-to-day, she has a strong spirit. She has a great support group of friends and family and her faith in God. HELLO GORGEOUS! is performing a wonderful service to women going through cancer treatment; I wish the group had been available when I was going to treatment. It is so good to feel normal even for a little while. A huge thanks to Kim, Trisha and Mike also, who works behind the scenes to make it all happen. Please continue this mission. God bless you all.

Marilyn

Shortly after we had Cindy's visit, she called me because she loved, loved, loved the wig that I had given her. The ones that she had were quite uncomfortable. The wig we had gotten her was so comfortable that she had forgotten she had it on and bent over her oven at home when she was baking and melted the front of her wig! She called us back in a panic and wanted to know if there was any way that we could get another wig, the same exact color and style, so that she could look the same as she had before. So that's quite a testament to the products that we use and that have been gifted to us.

# Cindy's Update

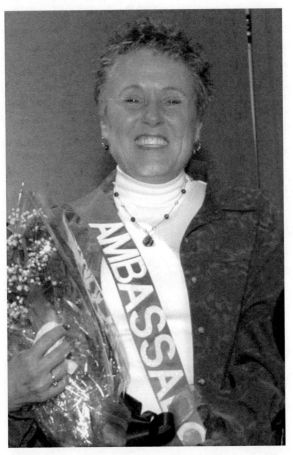

Cancer is an event in a woman's life unlike any other; there is loss of what is familiar in one's own body and spirit. Your body changes, your emotions are on a roller coaster and the semblance of ordinary life is shattered.

I was blessed throughout the time of my illness with faithful friends, a loving family and strength from God. My association with Hello Gorgeous! was life-changing in that the physical experience was not only mentally uplifting but I met Kim and Trisha, who have become wonderful friends. Each time I share my awesome day with a friend, I not only tear up but smile at the wonderful memories. I cherish the opportunity that I had in being the recipient of their loving services and, now that I am the 2011 Gorgeous! Ambassador for Hello Gorgeous! I hope to assist in gaining awareness for the Hello Gorgeous! Program.

# Kathy

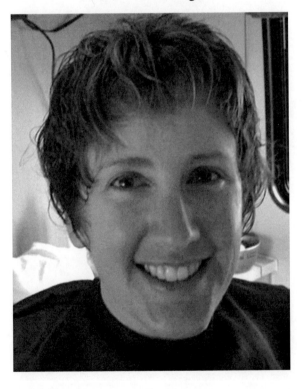

## "Trust Your Instincts"

Hello Gorgeous!

KATHY WAS ONE OF THE FIRST WOMEN done in the mobile Day-Spa. She was diagnosed with a rare cancer and endowed with a brave and persevering heart. Here is her story in her own words:

"I felt a lump in my breast in December 2008. I had no history of cancer in my family so I wasn't too worried about it, but knew that I should do my due diligence and have it checked out. My daughter, Allison, was 14 months old at the time, so I had a very special reason to be responsible about it. I waited until after Christmas and went to see my doctor in January. She sent me for a mammogram right away, but also said that she didn't think we needed to be too worried about it. The mammogram and ultrasound was a day or two later. The doctor came in after they were done and told me that I had very dense breast tissue and that there was nothing there. I tried to explain that there was a new lump, but he convinced me that there was nothing there and that I should start taking birth control pills to see if that helped. That was my first mistake. I should have INSISTED that the doctor do an exam and FEEL what I was trying to explain to him. But instead, he never touched me. He told me what I wanted to hear and I accepted it. The lesson here is to trust your instincts and demand that you get proper care. Perhaps my story would be much less complicated if that day had gone differently.

Instead I started taking the birth control pill and watched the lump get bigger for three months, all the while telling myself that it was nothing. At the urging of my husband, Ryan, I finally called my doctor back and told her what was going on. After an ultrasound, MRI, and two biopsies, I was diagnosed with angiosarcoma in my breast, which is a very rare type of vascular cancer. I had a mastectomy right away and was cancer-free! The cancer had not spread anywhere else. What a relief! The doctor recommended six months of weekly chemotherapy, then radiation, to make sure the cancer did not come back.

Hello Gorgeous! surprised me during my last week of chemotherapy, in October 2009. I was in total shock!

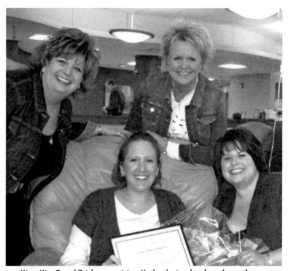

Kim, Kim Z and Trisha surprising Kathy during her last chemotherapy

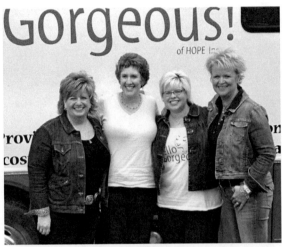

Kim, Kathy, Trisha and Kim Z

I had heard a little about them, but never dreamed that I was worthy of their services. In fact, I was a little uncomfortable with all the attention! I went on to have six weeks of radiation and, by this time, Christmas was upon us. We were all so busy that I didn't arrange to have my makeover until May 2010. Hello Gorgeous! showed up in front of my house in their mobile DaySpa and my morning of beauty began. By that time, a few inches of my hair had grown back and Kim was able to highlight it. I was so excited! I was pampered with a facial, manicure and pedicure, a haircut and highlights. What a wonderful reward for all that I had been through the year before! And spending the morning with Kim and Trisha, two of the most amazing women you will ever meet, was more than I could ask for. They made me feel so special."

# Kathy's Update

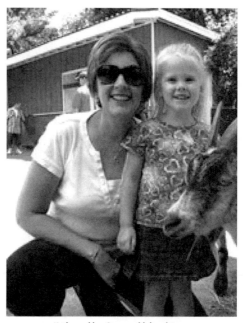

Kathy and her 3-year-old daughter

In November 2010, I found out that the cancer had returned . . . this time to the bones in my pelvis. I am currently undergoing chemotherapy. My daughter is now three years old and I am determined that I will win this battle for her. We have a beautiful little family, filled with a lot of love, and I will not allow cancer to take that away from us. I don't know where I will end up when this journey is over, but I believe I have a purpose here on earth and that cancer will show me just what that purpose is.

# Elise

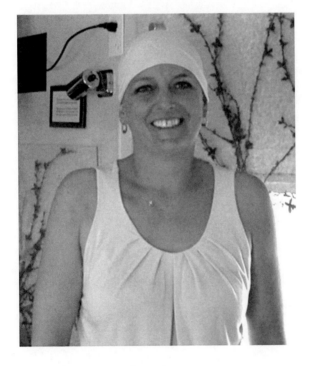

## "I should be on the other side of the TV"

Hello Gorgeous!

ELISE WAS OUR LAST GORGEOUS VISIT on the six-week tour in 2010. Nominated by a coworker, her afternoon of shopping turned into the afternoon of her life. Here's her story in her own words:

> On May 6, 2010, my world changed in ways that I could not have anticipated. The surgeon called me with the results from the biopsy he had taken from my lymph nodes near my left collar bone. He gently, but clinically, told me, "You have Hodgkin's Lymphoma."
>
> Before I could wrap my head around this diagnosis, I was referred to an oncologist for tests every day of the week except one to stage the cancer. I then knew from the results that I was at Stage III and a chemotherapy cocktail of ABVD would be the next course of action. All this was the result of my not getting over sinusitis and accidentally feeling a small, hard lump in the lower part of my neck.
>
> In an instant, I was on a path that amplified the unknowns that life brings since birth. I dealt with this dreaded news by making it as okay as I possibly could by calling my therapist, finding another oncologist I could have a working relationship with during this treatment process, and continuing in earnest the questions I had about my life's purpose.

After a port was surgically implanted in my chest, the liquid chemicals were infused into my body to help keep it on this Earth a while longer. I would have the treatment 12 times to conquer the multiplying cancer cells. The chemo would build in my body and no one could tell me the effects because everyone reacts differently, except for the hair loss.

Just before my third treatment, I shaved my head. Hair had started to come out in clumps like a shedding dog and I decided when all would be gone, before the treatment of the lymphoma told me this timetable as well. The changes that take place with one's body can be disheartening and it is a lonely process.

Less than a week after my third chemotherapy treatment, dear friends of mine told me we were going out for lunch. The value of these times, however simple, when people I loved reached out to me, cannot be overstated. Yet this time would be a whole lot different, unbeknownst to me.

On July 18th, I was not quite sure why my three amigas were being so mysterious, but it was made clear rather quickly. We arrived at a JC Penney store and I saw a couple more friends. Something told me it was not a coincidence, but what the heck could it be?

All of a sudden, I hear, "Hello Gorgeous! Elise Nothstine!!"

A small group of people came rushing toward me while even more people watched as they parted the way. Two children with big smiles earnestly thrust flowers and candy while letting

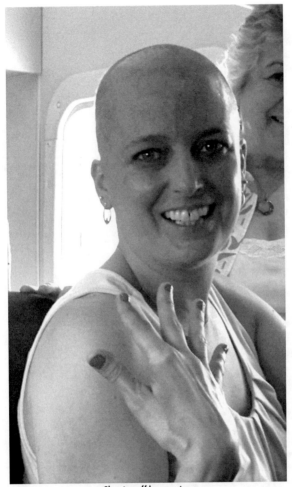
Showing off her manicure

me know they were for me. For me?! Whatever could they mean?

Little did I know that one of my friends from work who had mysteriously shown up at the store had learned about Hello Gorgeous! from a South Bend news show and had nominated me for a makeover. She had taken the time to make the contacts and explain why she felt I deserved such a treat. And now to my amazement, I was about to be the recipient of such a makeover that would beautify my outside and fill me with love and gratitude on the inside.

I kept thinking and would continually say throughout the day, "I should be on the other side of the TV!" Now I had read or heard about something like this happening to others, but this had now joyfully become my experience when I needed it most.

With my head wrapped in a scarf, I was whisked to the waiting mobile salon. I received a manicure, pedicure, and facial for the first time in my thirty-eight years of life. A wig that was thoughtfully trimmed now replaced the scarf and

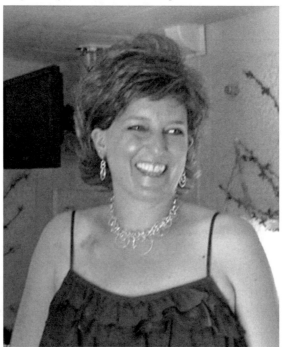

Elise after

I was graciously given a complete outfit of my choosing while being pampered for the day.

I had humbly thought this was the end of a day that was imprinted on my heart, but once again I was fooled. Then I was taken away with my new-found Hello Gorgeous! friends to an undisclosed destination for more generosity. We arrived at a local TGIF restaurant where Zumba dancers were rocking the music with flushed faces. They had not stopped moving until our arrival. What more could there possibly be in this most perfect day?

The instigator of my Hello Gorgeous! make-over had invited more friends from work to share this time by having lunch and celebrating life. In particular, my life with newly painted red nails and an outfit that helped me forget the changes cancer had brought to my body.

I could be quoted as saying that "just because I had worn Underoos, it did not make me Wonder Woman!" I highly suspect that everyone that made that day so special all had some superhero undergarments on to be so amazing and make that day so powerful that it will last a lifetime. And now with remission under my imaginary magic lassoed belt, I can gratefully say, "Hello Gorgeous!" with a whole new meaning.

# Elise's Update

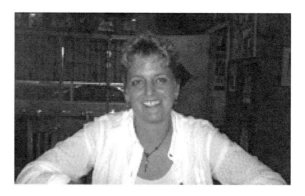

My update, as of August 2, 2011, is six months in remission! I've still got my port for chemo infusions as a precaution because the first two years are the highest risk for recurrence and I will have it for another 1½ yrs. I'm still kickin' and don't anticipate pushin' up daisies any time soon :) Wahoo! Thanks for everything! I hope our paths cross soon.

# Sue

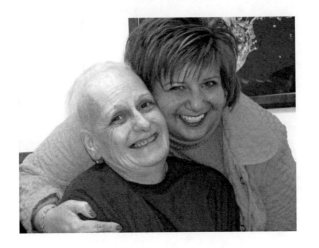

# "You Made Me Feel
So Special!"

# Hello Gorgeous!

I WANT YOU TO MEET MY FAVORITE AUNT. (She will tell you that she is my *only* aunt.) My Aunt Sue. Aunt Sue is my mom's sister. She and I have always been close, but then we got a little bit closer.

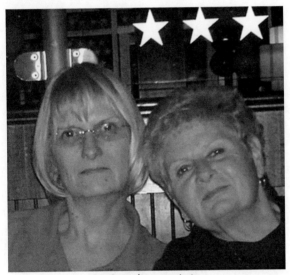

Aunt Sue and my mom, Janice

In December 2008 Aunt Sue was diagnosed with breast cancer. The tumor was the size of a grapefruit. The doctor had decided to do chemo first to shrink the tumor, then surgery to remove what they could, then radiation to make sure it was gone.

My Michael went to every chemo appointment with her, sat and held her hand. And I did what I knew how to do. I cut her hair into a short style so that it would ease some of the pain when it started falling out. I then called my friend and mentor Gloria and arranged for Aunt Sue to get a wig. I worked with her to show her how to draw her eyebrows on and found some really cute bangs that we cut to shape around her face that could be worn under her comfy terry cloth turban.

Aunt Sue never let me shave her head. She was more comfortable keeping whatever she could of her own hair.

In April, after she was diagnosed, I asked Aunt Sue if she would help us tell the story of Hello Gorgeous! We wanted to produce a storyboard with pictures that would depict what Hello Gorgeous! is all about, who we were and what we did.

We met at the salon on the Saturday before Easter. I asked her to bring a change of clothes and her smile. We took pictures to show what an actual Hello Gorgeous! visit would be like. We would manicure one of Aunt Sue's hands, take the pictures that we needed, and then quickly paint the second hand to match. Same with the pedicure—we performed the pedicure on one foot, quick pictures, then painted the other toes to match. When it came to the facial, we applied the mask, took the pictures to tell the story, then took the mask off. We applied Aunt Sue's makeup, had her change clothes and took some more photos. Her smile that day was radiant.

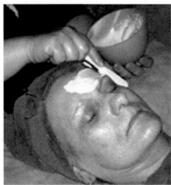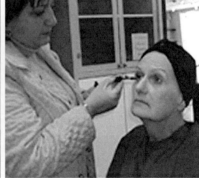

Aunt Sue's day of semi-pampering

The next day was Easter Sunday and we met at my mom's for Easter dinner. When Aunt Sue saw me she came up to me and gave me a huge hug and said, "Thank you for making me feel so special yesterday."

"Are you kidding me?" I said. "We violated you!" She told me that she lay in bed that morning just thinking about the day before and how much fun she had with us. Aunt Sue later admitted to me that she left the polish on her toes for six months. Every time she looked down and saw the polish color, it reminded her of her special day.

In August of 2009 Aunt Sue was declared in remission and is still cancer free today. Aunt Sue is a true inspiration.

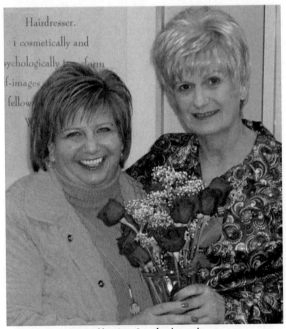

Kim and her Aunt Sue after her makeover

She fought this battle with poise and dignity and used this experience to empower. She went back to school and completed an associate degree in accounting, something she had always wanted to do. She was our very first Gorgeous! Ambassador and one of our biggest advocates for Hello Gorgeous! and for Mike and I.

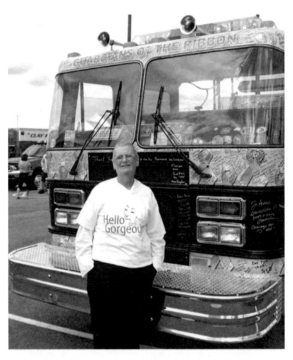

Sue visiting the pink fire truck and the sentiment she left

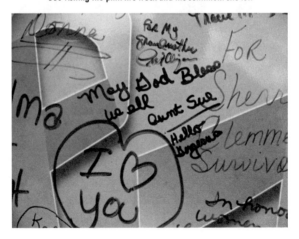

# Phyllis

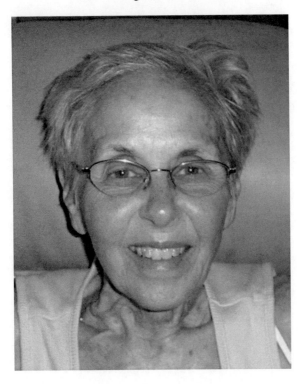

## "An Angel in Heaven"

Hello Gorgeous!

PHYLLIS WAS DIAGNOSED WITH MESOTHELIOMA and telling her story is her wonderful daughter, Pam:

I have never met a woman that had a deeper faith in God or a bigger fighting spirit than my Mom, Phyllis. She was diagnosed with Mesothelioma in February of 2008. Mesothelioma is a cancer that is caused by exposure to asbestos. We may never know how she was exposed to asbestos as the latency period (the time from first exposure to manifestation of disease) is prolonged and can be up to 30-40 years. All my family knows is that we now have an angel in heaven that we were lucky to once have in our lives and we miss her every single day.

After the initial shock of her diagnosis wore off, I remember thinking, "My mother has never smoked, rarely drank alcohol, and she was now being diagnosed with a terminal illness?" Doesn't seem quite fair, does it? She never complained. Not once. In fact, when learning of her fate, she said in her typical semi-sarcastic fashion, "Well, if I would have known that this is what I would end up with, I would have lived it up a little more." Fortunate for most, including my own mother, we do not know our fate which is why we should all strive to live each day like our last and give back to others daily.

I could write an entire book on the lessons that my mother taught me about life, relationships and faith. Being the mother of five children, she always had a lot of lessons that she was learning as well. I can rarely find the exact words to describe what an amazing mother my mom was and how blessed I was to have her in my life. She encouraged togetherness, strength in family, fighting battles like her cancer straight on...no backing down. She was very vocal about not being afraid to die even when the rest of us feared losing her daily.

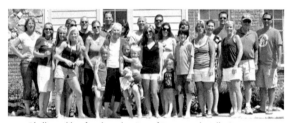

Phyllis and her family on her Day of Beauty with Hello Gorgeous!

My mom, Phyllis, passed away on March 9, 2011, but her legacy—wise words, devotion to her family and smile—will live on forever. My Mom grew up in a time when moms stayed home with their children; so consequently, all five of us children were with my mom a lot. Lucky us! She also worked at a high school in Fort Wayne, Indiana, for 32 years and we willingly shared her as a mom daily. She loved children and guiding them through life, and she did it well.

The gift that Hello Gorgeous! of Indiana gave to my mother was more than just making her beautiful for a day. In the midst of the ugliest disease in the world (cancer), my mom could feel like a normal woman again. No chemo, no pills, no dull skin or hair loss. Who knew that such a simple act of kindness could boost the morale of a woman with cancer and make her feel like a queen!

Hello Gorgeous! of Indiana is a blessing from God and from all the women who are victors and from those who lost the fight . . . THANK YOU, Kim and Mike Becker and all the Hello Gorgeous! family!

When we contacted Pam about writing her mother's story for this book, she also asked her father John to write for it as well. John took care of Phyllis as she fought her cancer and he kept all their family and friends updated periodically as to her condition with his profound words of love and understanding.

*Dear Pam:*

*Your words in reference to your mother are from your heart. . . . How can you improve on words that are so beautiful and adequate?*

*Your mother was and is a very special woman. I, for one, can never find the words that can ever fully express my love for her. She was like that... a woman so very much loved by all who knew her.*

*A woman who gave us all an image of herself that will overflow with our love for her eternally—and stamp her caring love forever on our souls.*

*Love, forever.*

   Your father

# Phyllis's Update

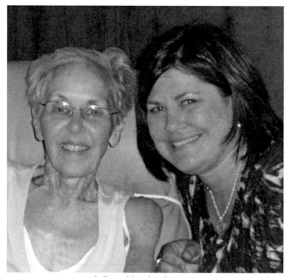

Phyllis and her daughter, Pam

Phyllis lost her battle with cancer on March 9, 2011. She was an exceptional woman and, although we had never met before our Gorgeous Day together, I could glimpse the depths of her humanness and her soul through the love and devotion of her family. And knowing all that I am because of the love and teaching I received from my own mother through my life, I understand Abraham Lincoln's words:

> "All that I am, or hope to be,
> I owe to my angel mother."

# Shelly

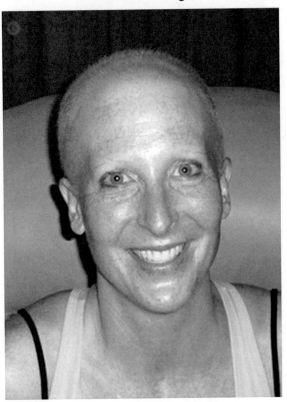

## "Thanks for the Mammaries!"

# Hello Gorgeous!

SHELLY IS A ZUMBA INSTRUCTOR that we kidnapped off a zumba stage in the middle of a shopping mall. Shelly was diagnosed with breast cancer, went through chemotherapy, radiation and a double mastectomy. Shelly was very positive throughout her battle and has a very supportive, loving husband and family.

It was Shelly's visit that caused a different vision in the Hello Gorgeous! program. Our original ideas for the Hello Gorgeous! Experience included the notion that these women would want services done in a private environment, far from the public and their prying eyes. We thought they would enjoy that cloistered environment, but we could not have been much further from the truth.

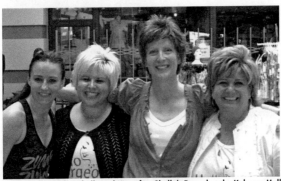

Zumba Kelly, Trisha, Shelly and Kim after Shelly's Reveal at the Kokomo Mall

When we constructed the plan to hold this event at the mall in Kokomo, Indiana, Shelly was under the impression that she was at the mall for a "Zumbathon" to benefit herself, as she was going through treatment at the time. Zumba is a Latin-inspired fitness dance program that is very popular now. And if you could have seen the look on her face while, during the second song of the day, with her dancing away, we marched up onto the stage and presented her with candy and flowers and told her that we were going to treat her to a day of beauty! The marketing director at that mall sent a note to all of the retailers there about who we were, notifying them of what was going to take place.

Once Shelly was in the DaySpa, over the course of the next three hours, a dozen or so retailers came knocking on

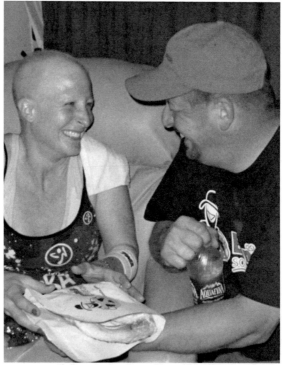

Shelly getting her treasured pretzel from Mark

the door of the Mobile DaySpa requesting to see Shelly and presented her with a gift. She was gifted a pair of shoes, shower gel and body lotion, a pearl bracelet and necklace, a new outfit, a "foofy" coffee drink and (the hit of the day since she was *STARVING!*) was a pretzel from Ben's Soft

Pretzels. You could not wipe the smile off of Shelly's face! This is when we realized that these amazing women do not want to be left alone. *They spend too much time alone.* People don't know what to say to people struck with cancer, so they say nothing and they stay away. Our program took on a new life, thanks to Shelly, and the Affiliate program was born. We designed a program that would be taken back into the salons across the United States, to take care of these courageous women on a regular basis in their own communities.

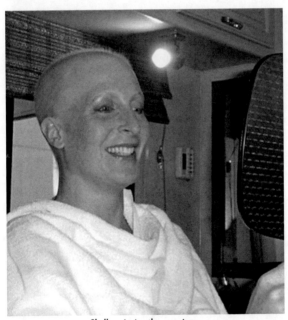
Shelly enjoying the experience

Shelly is truly an inspiration and a woman who embraced her disease and used it for good. When her double mastectomy was performed, she had someone take a picture of her in the hospital from her neck to her belly button and posted it to a popular social networking site with a caption that read:

"If this doesn't encourage you to get your mammogram, I'm not sure what will."

When I asked Shelly if she was considering reconstruction surgery, her response was, "No, I think I will just get a tattoo across my chest that says 'thanks for the mammaries'!"

Shelly is truly a marvelous woman and I draw my strength from her and others like her.

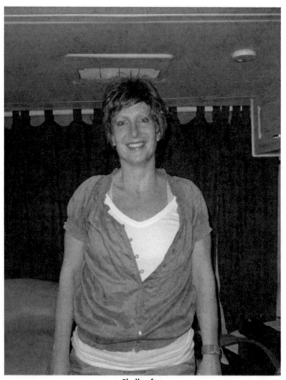

Shelly after

## Shelly's Update————————————————

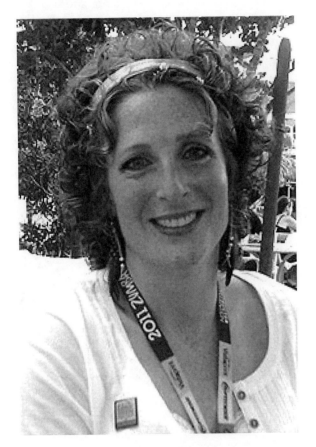

I am one year out of treatment and I am feeling more and more like myself every day. I have to finish my Herceptin treatments. Thankfully, I have no real lasting side effects. I look at pictures of myself before cancer and I don't rec- ognize that person anymore. I evolved, by God's plan, into a different person—seeing life more clearly and also the gifts that I have been blessed with in my life. I have a loving, devoted husband who carried me through cancer, sometimes on his shoulders. I have parents who have gladly taken the burden of cancer from me. I have a twin who never missed an appointment (well...until golf season started!). I understood my older sister's fight with MS more clearly. I saw what a wonderful brother I actually have. And, of course, my INCREDIBLE supportive network of friends! Now, I have you guys to thank for making me feel like a woman again. Hello Gorgeous! knew exactly what I needed when I needed it! Your mission is truly a Godsend. You will never know the impact you have had on my life, as well as countless others.

I look forward to today and hope for tomorrow.

Shelly

# Tracey

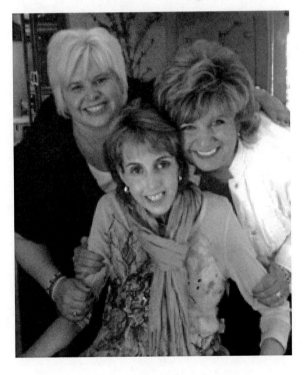

## Our Inspiration

## Hello Gorgeous!

IN MAY OF 2010 WE WERE ASKED TO participate in the Susan G. Komen Walk for a Cure. The organizers asked if we would be willing to award a visit to a breast cancer survivor for this event. We serve all women with all cancers, but for this event we decided to comply.

We received a nomination for Tracey from Warsaw, Indiana. Tracey had been diagnosed in March of 2005 with breast cancer. Tracey was unable to attend the race that year so we presented her award to her team and they we so excited for her. We decided to make Tracey our first stop on our tour that summer—that was until I received a phone call from Tracey's mother-in-law, Dixie. Dixie explained to us that Tracey wasn't doing well and asked if we could move the date of Tracey's visit up. I spoke with Trisha and we decided to make the visit happen the Sunday of Memorial Day weekend. Dixie was very appreciative.

We arrived at Tracey's home in Warsaw, Indiana, and pulled the Mobile DaySpa right up in front of her house and rolled the red carpet out onto Tracey's front lawn. We readied the bus to give Tracey a perfect day and waited patiently for Tracey to come out of the house and down the red carpet.

It was explained to us that Tracey, overnight, had lost her ability to walk, so Tracey's husband and brother-in-law carried Tracey from the house to the bus using a bag chair. We got her into the Mobile DaySpa and got her as comfortable as she could be. Tracey was in a lot of pain. But Tracey and I made a pact: I would stop asking her if she was okay, as long as she would tell me when she wasn't. It was agreed and we proceeded with her day of beauty—a facial, manicure, pedicure, highlights, blow dry and flat iron and we did Tracey's makeup.

Julie, Tracey's close friend, also spent the day with us. Julie is also a breast cancer survivor. They shared the story of how they had met and then Julie shared with us that Tracey had been a helicopter pilot in the United Stated Navy and showed a picture to us of Tracey and her chopper.

We shared laughs and no tears. I had acquired some information about Tracey's likes and dislikes in clothes. So I went shopping for Tracey and picked out a couple of things for her to choose from. Then we helped Tracey change into her new clothes.

Unbeknownst to Tracey, I had suggested to her family that they invite a few a friends to celebrate Tracey's new look. So little by little we watched as people filtered into Tracey's backyard. She kept asking what was going on. We just told her to mind her own business and enjoy the rest of her makeover.

When we finished with Tracey's makeover her husband and brother-in-law returned to the Mobile DaySpa with the bag chair to carry Tracey back into the house. Julie had invited us into the house to celebrate also. As we walked up the front sidewalk we heard a resounding "Hello Gorgeous!" and a huge applause from the backyard. There were so many people there to show their love to Tracey! We stayed for just a few minutes and watched all of the smiles that surrounded her.

I walked over to Tracey to give her a big hug and to say goodbye. We told each other "I love you" and I told her to get better fast.

When I left that house that day there was not a doubt in my mind that I would see Tracey at our big fundraiser in November. Her will to live and determination to fight this horrible disease was awe inspiring. She was a remarkable woman.

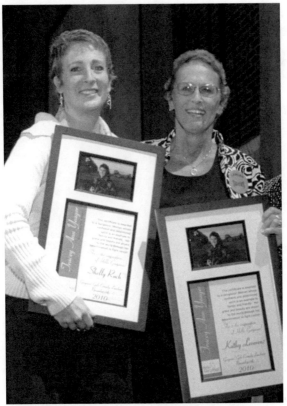

Shelly and Kathy, winners of the 2010 Tracey Yeager Award

We performed Tracey's visit on Sunday of Memorial Day Weekend. On Tuesday June 1st we received a phone call that Tracey had lost her battle against breast cancer on Memorial Day. She had died the day after our visit with her.

I was in shock. The news of Tracey's passing hit me like

a ton of bricks. I had thought that, as strong as her will was, losing that battle wasn't even an option for Tracey. I later spoke with a family friend who told me that the night of our visit with Tracey, as her husband was putting her to bed, she said to him, "I know this sounds crazy, but today was one of the best days of my life."

We have established an inspirational award in Tracey's name that will be given to a special Gorgeous! Woman each year in November at our Comedy Luncheon. I had the pleasure of knowing Tracey for only a very short period of time but I am forever changed by her will to fight and her determination to live. She is a true inspiration.

# HOPE

# hope (houp)

*v.*

1. To wish for something with expectation of its fulfillment.
2. Something which one longs to see realized.
3. The virtue by which a Christian looks with confidence for God's grace in this world and glory in the next.

# One Definition of HOPE

First of all, our name has the word HOPE in it. The "hope" in Hello Gorgeous! of HOPE, Inc. stands for:

**H**elping

**O**thers

**P**ersevere

**E**veryday

and this is truly what we attempt to do every day. And I can tell you that, while normal people take it for granted that they will wake up tomorrow and that their days of living stretch out endlessly before them, those battling cancer are very conscious of each and every day they live. Their HOPE is to persevere until tomorrow—two very different views of life and living.

This definition does not refer to the amazing stories you've just read. As Mike and I reminisce over our experiences with the women in this book, we see all of these women as examples of excellence and character, of what is best in the human spirit. That is what we have seen every day working with these women.

But the hope that we speak of here is that *more* of these women can be helped in this critical way, with the Hello Gorgeous! Experience: tens of thousands, rather than hundreds. So Hello Gorgeous! has taken a step toward making this happen.

In the summer of 2010 our family packed for a 6-week trip and began a twenty-city tour of Indiana. We prearranged and surprised 20 women battling cancer. We gifted them with a complete makeover and Revealed them to a group of their friends and family in a public setting. Our purpose was to introduce our concept to other communities in Indiana and the response was wonderful. But after 40 days on the road, in our 18th hotel, we realized that enough women were not being helped. And if Hello Gorgeous! remained only three people and a mobile DaySpa, even on the road 50 weeks a year, enough women never would be. You see, there are over 30,000 women each year diagnosed with cancer in Indiana alone; 700,000 nationwide; and that does not count all those women from the previous year that are still in treatment. A hundred women helped a year is not enough. We needed to do more.

And so on the road we began to design the *Affiliate Salon Program*, a certification for salon owners and stylists in existing salons, in cities across the United States. It outlines how to perform the Hello Gorgeous! Experience in their own salons, bringing this service to women battling cancer in their own communities, a service that would stay in their community as well.

We chose talented, experienced salons in these communities for this program and, as they are top professionals, we need not show these stylists how to perform manicures or pedicures. What we demonstrate is how to perform these services on women with cancer; those people experiencing risks and challenges with their immune system. These are subtle but important differences.

The Hello Gorgeous! formula is based on three E's:

- ❖ we create an Experience;
- ❖ that Empowers these women;
- ❖ by Educating them on how to manage the effects of their image trauma left behind by radiation and chemotherapy.

Like all cosmetologists, I went to beauty school. For the next 25 years after graduation, I was constantly focused on keeping up with the latest trends and education in our industry. This type of information was never talked about and, as far as I know, information and techniques to help women correct the image effects of their cancer treatments are still not in the curriculum today.

The broader vision of Hello Gorgeous! (through our website and our work in salons and in the beauty school system across the United States) is to inspire the up-and-coming youth in the beauty industry on these techniques so that, armed with this information, they will be able to help women who also *are not* in the Hello Gorgeous! Program: clients, friends and family that have their own cancer challenges and questions. It is all about helping the women.

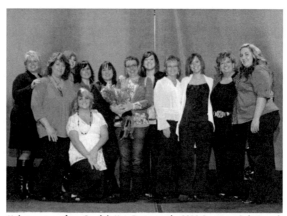

Makeover team from Sandy's Hair Design at the 2010 Gorgeous Gals Comedy Luncheon and their Gorgeous Woman, Lynn. What a great day!

This picture is of Kim, Trisha and our first Affiliate Salon, *Sandy's Hair Design of South Bend, IN*, posing with the Gorgeous Woman they had the privilege to make over at an event last year. Sandy, the owner of the salon, confided to us after the event how working with women battling cancer had changed them and bonded their team. It changed me as well.

It changes what you worry about in your life. When you spend three hours with a woman whose thoughts are: "I need to live long enough for my daughter to graduate from high school," it is difficult for you to worry about petty things like "who stole my Lean Cuisine out of the freezer" or "my kids left the house a mess." The idea of what is truly important in your life is tested.

# Here is a list
# of our fabulous Affiliate Salons
(so far):

Sandy's Hair Design, South Bend, IN
The Beehive, South Bend, IN
Bangs Salon and Spa, South Bend, IN
Nicholas J Salon and Spa, Notre Dame, IN
Creative Edge Hair Studio, Mishawaka, IN
FIX Spa Salon, Elkhart, IN
The Beauty Shoppe, Elkhart, IN
Expressions Day Spa, Warsaw, IN
Rain Salon and Spa, Noblesville, IN
Chateau Bijou, Noblesville, IN
CC Hair Company, Plymouth, IN
Michelle's Headquarters, Culver, IN
Studio 21, Gurnee, IL
Aqua Salon, Chicago, IL
Alternative Spa and Salon, Corry, PA
Aspasia Salon and Spa, St. Charles, MN
Studio She, Frederick, MD
On Purpose Hair Salon, Fort Wayne, IN

## Other amazing businesses that have helped Hello Gorgeous! with women battling cancer:

A Thousand Words Photography

Maurice's

Beauty Systems Group

Hoosier Racing Tires

Dress Barn

Mary Kay Cosmetics

Crowe Horwath LLC

Classic Image Photography

Chick-fil-A

JC Penney

Simon Properties

Macy's

Country Florist and Gifts

TGI Friday's

Applebee's

NIPSCO

Diane Shoemaker, CPA

Mark Borst and Cheveux Hair Salon